Table Manners
For Massage Therapists

How to Build an Excellent Practice

Mary Alice Walter, LMT

A Simple Prayer

Lord make me an instrument of your peace
Where there is hatred...let me sow love.
Where there is injury...pardon.
Where there is discord...unity.
Where there is doubt...faith.
Where there is error...truth.
Where there is despair...hope.
Where there is sadness...joy.
Where there is darkness...light.
O Divine Master, grant that I
May not so much seek
To be consoled...as to console.
To be understood as understand.
To be loved...as to love.
For it is in giving that we receive.
It is in pardoning that we are pardoned.
It is in dying that we are born to eternal life.

St. Francis of Assisi

To Erin and Kevin

Who give my life meaning

Acknowledgements

God has blessed me often throughout life and especially during this particular stage. For that I am very grateful. Many thanks also to Pam who went with me to SHI to see about enrolling in massage school when I had no idea if this was the right thing to do. Thank you for your friendship, then and always.

Thank you to everyone who taught me so much about the wonderful world of massage, in school and in practice, including Debbie Bomkamp, Tina Holsapple, Mary Cheers, Donna Busse, the late Peggy Allen, Staci Loer Fischer, Jennifer Larsen, Kathi Swango Klein, Rita Hopper, Ann Weber, Laura Lander, Gary McCarthy, and the staff at SHI Integrative Medical Massage School.

This book would never have happened without the expert and compassionate input of my editors and advisors Susan Unes, Ann MacKenzie, Kirk MacKenzie, Beth Staggenborg, and John Loughmiller.

I appreciate all of your contributions. Be Well.

Table of Contents

Introduction

"Every day remind yourself of your own ability, of your good mind, and affirm that you can make something really good out of your life."
Norman Vincent Peale

Congratulations on choosing the field of massage therapy. I hope you find it as fulfilling as I have for the last eleven years. It can be everything you dream for your work and your life if you understand what it takes to build a successful practice. There are many ways to approach and experience the daily requirements of being a successful therapist. You can have all the best intentions of making an honest effort at this and still have your ultimate dreams remain a bit out of reach. My hope is that by sharing with you the details of the thought processes I have gone through in my many years of dealings with clients and other therapists, you will have more keys in your pocket to make it happen for yourself.

Part One describes the "why" portion of what we do and how it affects those around us. It examines the elements of practice that you may not have considered, but these elements contribute everything to the comfort of your clients. And why do you want your clients to be comfortable with you? So they'll come back to you and bring their friends and family!

Part Two includes the "how" portion with specific examples of the kinds of activities you need to consider in order to create excellence in the practice of your dreams. How do you make your practice more inviting and effective? It is in the multitude of decisions you make, such as: where you will work, the types of clients you will work on, and how you will conduct yourself along the way. My hope is that *Table*

Manners will inform, inspire, and amuse you while building your confidence in your own worth and ability.

There is so much more to running a successful practice than effective treatment of injuries and aches. Throughout these pages we will discuss a multitude of details that can make all the difference in your clients' comfort. For example, if you talk all through the session and your client was looking for an hour of quiet and stillness, how likely is she to come back even if you made her shoulder feel better? Or how comfortable will a new client be if she gets on your table and finds your linens badly wrinkled, leading her to wonder if they are clean?

Whether you are still in massage school, newly licensed, or an experienced therapist, you will find suggestions, ideas, and encouragement here that can help you realize your dreams of becoming a successful therapist.

Massage schools, like most educational programs, teach all they possibly can in the time they have you in the classroom. As you probably are aware, however, the real learning in most professions often begins once you take that huge leap of faith out of the security of the classroom into the realm of actually serving clients.

Be happy in your work and remain committed to that happiness. You alone control your own happiness by the choices you make every day. By consciously and thoughtfully making the right choices for YOU each day, your work can be a great source of happiness, fulfillment, and prosperity as well as service to others.

I hope this book will help you build your practice more quickly by avoiding some of the most common mistakes of newbies or even experienced therapists. Believe me, I made all the mistakes in this book at least once! But I learned, turning each mistake into a lesson. By the grace of God many clients came back to see me and some became regulars, helping me to build a successful and mature massage practice. You can do this, I'm absolutely sure, because I did it and I consider myself fairly ordinary. I am a hard worker, though, and I was determined to make my practice a success for my own good and for the good of my clients. Make your practice your own, but don't bother reinventing the wheel. Let what I've learned sink in, consider it carefully, and take with you what makes sense to you. Watch your schedule fill, your confidence grow, and prosperity be yours in uncommon time. There are no limits to your success if you are willing to invest your time, energy, and attention toward positive progress.

Keep in mind some of these ideas may stretch you beyond your comfort zone. Be kind to yourself whenever you realize you are afraid. Replace all fear with love and watch your successes stack up. I was afraid of everything in the beginning! My excellent teachers told us we all would get comfortable with everything over time, and they were right. Now I look back over my progress and see that I've mastered many tasks that previously scared me, and I truly love my work. You will too, and I hope with the help of this book you will do it more quickly than I did. I understand how badly you want to be a success at this, because I've been there. I believe I can help you get to where I am now, which is working at a job I love every day and making a living in a fulfilling and peaceful career.

Confidence is an important element in success in most areas of life, and massage therapy is no different. Confidence may be even more important here! While it can take a lot of time to build confidence through experience, excellent training can boost that confidence significantly when we are just starting out. Some days you will feel like you can do anything, and other days you may feel like you can't do anything right! We've all been there! My goal is for you to feel much more confident in your abilities through reading the specific examples here and learning the finer details of being successful as a massage therapist. I was intimidated by everyone in the early days, and although I felt certain I was in the right place, I wasn't comfortable with choosing modalities for each client or asking them personal questions about their health. I decided to be my own encourager by taking one day and one task at a time and doing my best in every way possible. Slowly but surely I became more comfortable. I had good days where everything seemed possible, but the challenging days came far more often. The good days kept me going.

Here's an example of one good day early on: While in school and working on my practice clients, one friend agreed to let me practice my lessons on him. As a physician, he admitted he doesn't relax well and he told me right up front to not take it personally. He said he enjoys massage but he may not sound like he is relaxed as some people will. Well, this very same fellow went to sleep on my table during his first massage from me! That was a great boost to my confidence in the early days, and carried me through a lot of tough lessons. You'll have experiences like this too!

Every one of us is the result of choices we have made along the way. There are no exceptions. True, life has a way of 'happening' to us and often throws a curve ball. But whatever happens, you are in control of your response to each moment, each situation, and each challenge. If you don't like the result of your choices in the past, chalk up all those results to experience. Results are only considered failure if we fail to learn from them. The key to making new, better, healthier, productive choices that lead to your success is realizing you have this power, using it daily, and staying in the present moment as much as possible to choose wisely and create the success you desire.

Life in the wonderful world of massage therapy, as I like to call it, can be rewarding in so many ways. If you are like most people who become successful massage therapists, you have approached this field with a giving heart. Truly, that is the basis for success here, in my opinion. Massage therapy is therapy, which is giving, caring, looking out for your clients and patients. In the pages that follow, I will spell out the details that I have learned by making mistakes which ultimately taught me valuable lessons that I believe have contributed largely to my successful private practice.

Let's face it, there is a lot to learn already in the subjects of anatomy, physiology, massage modalities, hot and cold therapy, various ailments and treatments, and contraindications. It's very difficult for massage schools to spend much time on the psychology and professionalism of being an excellent therapist. This book is not an A&P book, nor is it a how-to of massage techniques. It is not a business book full of accounting tips or marketing strategies for running a business. The focus here is the psychology of excellence. It's about:

- How to take what you've learned in massage school as well as in life and add that to your dreams for your life as a massage therapist.
- Understanding how your attitudes have gotten you to where you are today and how they'll contribute to your future.
- Creating personal and authentic connections with clients and potential clients.
- Being aware and therefore being better able to make quality decisions daily that will bring you the success you desire without having to reinvent the wheel.
- Understanding what you and your clients are thinking so you can help them feel comfortable with you.

This book is designed so that you can read it all the way through from start to finish if you like, or you can open it at random and read a specific lesson. Focus your attention each day on something in particular you feel will help you be the best therapist possible. Knowing some of the best practices in the trade will give you an advantage in reaching a higher level of satisfaction with your new practice. You'll enjoy your work, feel confident in your knowledge and abilities more quickly, and produce an income that pays the bills quicker, allowing for a higher standard of living where you can save and spend more freely without worrying about every dime and every unfilled appointment. The reward for your clients is greater relief from discomfort and more effectively preventing future problems, which leads them to feel great and tell all their friends and co-workers about you.

If you are reading this book as a student or new therapist, enjoy this opportunity to side-step some of the struggles of therapists who have gone before you. You can learn from the solid experience of many people and go right to the tactics that have proven to be winners.

If you are reading this book as a practicing and successful massage therapist, you may be thinking, "I could have written this book." You are right! I'm sure you've found many ways to take good care of your clients and fulfill your right path. I hope as you read on that you will find encouragement for what you are already doing and continue to bring peace and healing to yourself and to all of your clients. In addition, I hope this book will inspire you to try a few new things, perhaps taking your practice to a new level of success. Maybe you'll become a mentor to a newer therapist in your area and share your passion and expertise with them.

Dr. Wayne Dyer said "The quality that stands out among those who feel inspired is a quality of intense, burning desire. The intensity of your desire needs to be so great that your love for who you are and what you do precludes the possibility of any boredom, tedium, or weariness."

We need more health, more peace, more compassion, and more love in this world. We as massage therapists share all of these things every day through our work. We need more excellent massage therapists who can encourage more clients/patients in their own quest for optimal health. Thank you for letting me share my thoughts and experiences with you.

A Little About Me...

I was in my mid-40s when I went to massage school. I previously had started and operated two successful businesses, worked many years for other people, and earned

18

a Bachelor's degree in Psychology as a part-time adult student. I raised two wonderful children to successful, self-sufficient independence. However, despite this amount of life experience, I quickly found out that I still had a lot to learn about making my massage practice stand out so that I would succeed again in this whole new area.

Here's the path I was on: being the third of seven siblings, six of which were girls, college was not an option when I was in high school. After graduation I got married and started a family. I enrolled in college part time when my daughter and son were both in grade school. It took me a full eleven years to complete my studies, during which time we moved twice and I got divorced. However, I graduated with honors at the age of 39, receiving a bachelor's degree in Psychology. When I was newly divorced I started my own full-time cleaning business. Being self-employed gave me the most flexibility to be available to my then young teenagers, and flexibility of schedule is still one of my top personal priorities. With my cleaning business the money was good, the respect was hard won and heartfelt, and the pace was acceptable; however the benefits, or lack of benefits, stunk – no paid vacation or sick days, no health insurance provided by an employer. Still, I felt it was worth it at the time.

Five years after the divorce I received my Bachelor's degree. By then I had changed jobs to working full time in a hospital laboratory with great benefits. I loved my job, the pay, my co-workers, and the health insurance, but I missed many events with my son and daughter. The flexibility I so preferred was completely gone. That hurt. For me, being a mom has always been my number one priority and the main purpose of my life. I stuck with the job though, until my position was eliminated in a merger. Although I lost my job I came away from this experience with a very valuable personal insight: I learned that one-on-one patient contact was something I enjoyed and was good at. The question now became how to put this new knowledge to good use in my next endeavor.

I found another job which put me in a leadership position. I loved the job and the people and thought it would be a job I could retire from someday. My long-term hopes came to an end after five years and I was again forced to figure out what to do next. By this time my daughter had graduated from college and gotten married, and my son was in graduate school and engaged to be married, so I was on my own. I enrolled in a massage therapy program, not sure at all if this was the right step for me. I had more questions than answers. The most pressing question was 'Can I be successful, quickly and also long term, at this? How long will it take to build my practice enough to make a living as a massage therapist?' These are real and pressing questions for anyone needing to make a living, and fast!!

My first homework assignment for massage class was to work on someone, a friend or family member, massaging their hands and arms only. I felt a bit silly approaching my first practice client even though he is a good friend, but something magical happened the instant I began practicing my lessons. I knew beyond a shadow of a doubt that I was in the right place, doing the right thing, at the right time in my life. What a wonderful feeling! Were all my questions immediately answered? No way! But it was enough for me to know I was where I needed to be, on the right path.

Although my adult children no longer needed me on a daily basis, I still wanted the freedom that I'd had before when I was self-employed. I was in my mid-forties now. My life and work experience up to this date resulted in a great benefit to my dream of a successful massage practice: I knew a lot of people, and they knew a lot of other people.

Early in the massage program I wrote a letter announcing my new endeavor and requesting volunteers who would give me the honor of practicing my lessons on them without payment. I sent the letter to absolutely everyone I knew, and encouraged them to share it with people they knew.

The response I received was thrilling! I set up a schedule to work on two people every week, at the very least, usually even through breaks in classes. This was in addition to the number of practice clients required by the school, which was plenty. By the tenth month in school, with eleven months to go until graduation and licensing boards, my practice schedule was completely full right up to the date of taking the medical boards. The next clients I could book would be paying clients because by then I'd be a professional, a Licensed Massage Therapist.

All that extra practicing really paid off. I quickly became comfortable with each and every technique I learned in classes because I practiced each one so often. By the time I was able to charge real money for giving massage, I felt competent in knowledge and experience. When clients came to see me with aches or pains, I had already worked on similar cases. I wasn't overwhelmed with absolutely everything being new. I was completely comfortable with taking medical histories because I included it on the first visit with all my practice clients. The extra practice might have been the single most beneficial decision I made that jump-started my private massage therapy practice.

For Whom this Book is Intended

If you are still in massage school, my intention is to help you hit the ground running once you pass your licensing boards. You can do quite a bit to build your future practice even before graduation. Right now, while in school, I highly encourage you to set up a practice schedule starting today. Invite everyone you know to visit you for free massage. The more people you see and practice on, the more you will increase your skills and confidence. Regardless of where you end up working, use the suggestions in this book to shape your career with excellence and achieve success to match your dreams.

If you are newly licensed and trying to figure out how to get more clients right now, this book is designed to help you navigate the many seemingly small but ultimately very important decisions you need to make to help get you to where you want to be as a successful therapist. You may still need to give away some free massages, but examining your attitude, your style, your practice, and shaping them all with excellence, will help you increase the number of clients you see each week. I hope *Table Manners* will encourage you with its many ideas. Perhaps it will inspire you to be creative and add more of your own ways to connect with clients and build your practice more quickly.

If you are reading this book as an experienced therapist who is interested in boosting your success to a higher level, read on. *Table Manners* is designed to infuse your work with excellence, leading you to greater success and fulfillment. You have experience to draw from, so sometimes a bit of tweaking of your current daily activities is all that is needed to take your practice from just okay or good to completely excellent and quite fulfilling.

Massage Therapy as a Spiritual Practice

Finally, a close relationship with Jesus Christ and a life-long dedication to service are, in my opinion, both keys to a successful massage therapy practice. My faith assures me that God is always a loving presence. I believe He is blessing every one of us at all times. I pray for my clients daily. I ask for blessings for my client on the table. I find creative ways to include prayer for my clients. Every month as I send out my newsletter and I see the individual names I ask for God's blessings on every one of my clients plus their friends and family. I am happy to serve in honor of our Creator and Source of all that is good. The way I see it is everything I do, everything I have, and everything I am, are all thanks to Him. He is the ultimate healer! Keep Him close to you by talking with Him daily and listening for guidance. You will see blessings you didn't realize were even possible. A prayer I personally use frequently is: "Father, today I choose to put

You first. I acknowledge that without You, I can do nothing. With You, ALL things are possible! I invite You to have Your way in my life as I seek You first in all that I do in Jesus' name. Amen."

People are often unreasonable and self-centered.

Forgive them anyway.

If you are kind, people may accuse you of ulterior motives.

Be kind anyway.

If you are honest, people may cheat you.

Be honest anyway.

If you find happiness, people may be jealous.

Be happy anyway.

The good you do today may be forgotten tomorrow.

Do good anyway.

Give the world the best you have,

and it may never be enough.

Give your best anyway.

For you see, in the end, it is between you and God.

It never was between you and them anyway.

Mother Teresa

Part One

The Psychology of Excellence

You too are building a monument to the quality of your life every day you live. You do it in the way you do your job, treat a stranger, a neighbor, or a colleague. You do it in the way you keep your promises, care for your possessions, and groom your body. In a thousand small ways during a million mundane moments you are building a reputation for excellence or mediocrity. How you build is up to you, but how you will be remembered is determined by that choice. Make it well. You and you alone will choose whether your life will be a testament to integrity or a cautionary tale.

David Foster, *Accept No Mediocre Life*

Your Success is Up To You

Aristotle said, "We are what we repeatedly do. Excellence, therefore, is not an act but a habit." Developing the habit of excellence is not as difficult as it sounds. Simply spend one minute doing the very best you can, no matter what it is you are doing. Then when that minute is over, repeat the procedure. Before you know it, a habit is born. Remember daily that your success is up to you. You really do have a tremendous amount of power over your success and your future. Realizing this as a basic truth is a big step in getting where you want to go. You have the power to make things happen!

Because I knew early on that I wanted to go into private practice once I was licensed, I listened intently to experienced therapists and I received many helpful ideas while I was still a student. I learned even more the good old-fashioned way: through trial and error as a student and as a professional. If I can save you a few months or years' time getting your practice to excellent status, and save you a few clients (or a lot!) that might not return as you find your way in the early months, then we will both have succeeded.

This section is about having a mindset of excellence and understanding what excellence looks and feels like. It's about how that excellence comes across to your clients and what effect it can have on them. Maya Angelou said, "People may forget what you say or what you do, but they never forget how you made them feel." Taking time to consider how you as a therapist can affect the way your clients feel is an important element in building your excellent practice and succeeding long term.

This section describes how to think about everything you do and infuse your own style into it until you and your practice exude excellence and clients come to you from all around. I can tell you this is what worked for me. The reason I know it worked is that I never once had a sign in front of my practice indicating that my massage therapy practice was in the building. My practice was built entirely by referrals.

People will talk about how you treated them during their time with you. They will react to how you made them feel. They will notice if you seemed to really care about them or if you were in a hurry to move on with your day.

If your primary focus in the massage business is to make a huge income quickly, please hear this next statement with sincere respect: you'll save yourself a lot of time and aggravation by quitting right now and redirecting your energy into a field more appropriate for you.

However, if your focus is on serving others, there are no limits to the success you can achieve in massage therapy, and the money will come. There is gentleness in serving, kindness in looking out for others. Massage therapy is about giving of your time and talents. It is about serving others. It's about assisting people on their own path to health and well-being. It has also been said that the quickest way to achieve our goals is to help others achieve theirs. Serving is all about looking for ways to help other people. People respond very favorably to excellent attention to their health and well-being. As they call it in the business world, "good customer service" will help you win clients.

As beginners in any field we naturally are lacking in experience, but we can really make up for it in work ethic. Show up; be professional. Be compassionate and show your clients you care about their well-being. Andrew Carnegie said, "The average person puts only 25 percent of his energy and ability into his work. The world takes off its hat to those who put in more than 50 percent of their capacity, and will stand on its head for those few and far between souls who devote 100 percent." Be prepared to work hard, to put yourself 100% into your work, and you will reap the benefits. Focus on what you want, which is a successful massage practice, and work at it diligently every day. Don't try to get by with going halfway. Do it all, and do it well. I believe your character is more important than your talent, and in the beginning your character can make up for your still-developing talents. I like the way Dave

Ramsey put it in *More Than Enough*, "Work is doing it. Discipline is doing it every day. Diligence is doing it well every day." Are you giving it your all or are you sometimes going through the motions?

Excellence is not about perfection

Excellence is the goal. Perfection is not. Perfection isn't possible for anyone. I think Winston Churchill got it absolutely right when he said, "Perfectionism spells paralysis." Trying to be perfect can cause us to stand still and do nothing for fear of making a mistake, or be so nervous about doing everything "right" that we turn people off or end up completely frustrated. Aiming for excellence frees you to imagine success in whatever ways it makes sense to you and doesn't tie you down to doing everything "right". Because what is "right"? Making your practice excellent might not look the same as the next therapist's practice, and that is okay! Excellence is about being YOUR best! On the other hand, excellence is not about status and is never about gaining an advantage over another person. That is true for clients, family, friends, colleagues, and even strangers. Excellence isn't competing with colleagues and worrying about who has more clients per week. Excellence is being your best, whatever you are doing, and helping others achieve their own success too.

Keep your focus on this goal of an excellent practice, and make daily decisions based on investing your time and energy to that end. While the early days/weeks/months are less full with paying clients, more time is available for you to think about your practice and look for ways to make it professional, excellent, inviting, and uniquely your own. Do you believe you can be successful? You can! Believe it! Do you feel gratitude for every paying client that you have? Give thanks! Do you express your interest in the wellbeing of each client? Listen to them! Do you look for ways to help your clients, and potential clients, feel peaceful in your presence? The day-to-day details for creating excellence are in the next section. For now, let us focus on how to think about your needs and the needs of clients and what will help them see the excellence in you and in your practice.

While you have time between clients in the early days, think of ways to let everyone know that you are a professional, you are open for business wherever you are practicing, and you are ready to serve! On days less busy with clients, there are many ways to build your practice and lots of excellent decisions to be made:

- **Create your web site** and fill it with helpful information so prospective clients can find you, learn about you, and begin to become comfortable with you and your approach to massage therapy.
- **Decide on your menu of services** and prices and develop a brochure so readers understand whether you focus on sports massage, cancer massage, pregnancy massage, etc., and they can learn your fees and your schedule.
- If you are working for an established spa or the like, **learn all you can** about the business itself, any special products they offer, and any new techniques they want you to learn.
- **Consider marketing tools** like referral bonuses for existing clients such as 15 minutes free on their next massage when a friend or relative books a session with you. Consider offering a holiday special. Do you want to set a referral policy that rewards clients for bringing in friends which keeps clients coming back too? People love bargains and early on is the best time to utilize specials that make people happy to get a discount!
- **Research credit card companies** so you can be ready to make payment easy for clients and keep costs low for yourself.

- Open a **special checking account** for your practice so you can keep your finances in excellent professional order.
- Plan and host an **Open House**. Invite everyone to check out your new office space. Be sure to include a raffle for a few free massages. The winners will be delighted!
- **Develop a newsletter** to share helpful and healthful tips with your clients. The newsletter goes a long way in showing your clients that you care because you give it away, electronically or on paper, without charging them. Filling it full of healthful information allows you to show them again that you care about their health.
- Consider whether or not you want to use **social media** to help promote your practice.
- **Join the local business association**, if one is available, to meet other business owners in town and help them get to know you. Learn about local events in which your participation might cost a little time but little or no money. There is a lot of free marketing in taking time to get to know your neighbors.
- Read a few pages from your anatomy and physiology book to **stay knowledgeable**. Excellence!
- Exercise, stretch, meditate, and practice yoga to **build your strength and stamina** so you will be healthy and strong for your growing practice.
- Ask the universe: **"How may I serve today?"** Listen for answers and direction. Follow it!
- Schedule at least one hour per week for **dream time**. This is your hour to spend thinking about what you want and how your practice will look, feel, and smell when it is fully operational. Breathe in the feeling of success and satisfaction you will feel when you reach your goals. Feel it now!

All of these tasks take time, thought, effort, vision, and will be great investments in your future success. This is the time to get your ducks in a row so you'll be ready for clients when they do come! Many of these early decisions will set the stage for your practice and once they are accomplished your investment will pay off for years to come. In the beginning it may seem like you never get away from work. True, you will be totally immersed in thinking about work. This is a brief period, however, compared to the years your excellent practice will serve you and your clients once it is up and running. Many of the decisions you make now will not need to be reevaluated for quite a few years, so the work load will decrease as you check these decisions off the list. Many of these activities will bring in clients slowly and steadily. As your client numbers increase you will also build your physical strength, increase your people skills, and refine your massage approach. Over time your vision of becoming a successful massage therapist will materialize right before your eyes!

When I was a new therapist, one or two clients per day were plenty because I wanted time after each one to look up any muscle or medical issues they talked about. There was so much more to learn! I was happy to have the time to switch gears between clients and consider the massage techniques I chose for each one. Now I routinely give three to six massages in a day, often going right from one to the next with only 30 minutes between sessions. It takes time to build this kind of experience which leads to confidence. You'll get there, and the time invested up front will never be wasted. History shows us that Abraham Lincoln was a master at keeping focus on his goal. Author Daniel Goleman once spoke of Lincoln saying, "Having hope means that one will not give in to overwhelming anxiety, a defeatist attitude, or depression in the face of difficult challenges or setbacks. Hope is more than the sunny view that everything will turn out all right. It is believing you have the will and the way to accomplish your goals." As long as you have hope, you will be inspired to keep moving forward toward your dreams.

Vision and Values

Have a strong vision and examine your values to help you in deciding how you would like your massage practice to look and feel. Daydream when you take breaks from studying. Let your mind wander. See the details like actual decorations in your treatment room or your office space. Picture yourself talking with your ideal client. Who is it? An athlete? A cancer patient? An over-worked parent? The elderly? If you grew up in the company of a grandparent and are completely comfortable around the elderly, perhaps this is the population you would feel the most fulfilled to work with. On the other hand if you are or were an athlete, and you know exactly which muscles need attention for runners or ballplayers, maybe you will prefer sports massage. There are so many options available, not just in the massage world but in all of life. Considering what YOU value most will lead you to make right decisions FOR YOU. Choosing one doesn't mean the others are less valuable, they're just not the best for you. I firmly believe that if each of us carefully considers our own values and preserves them in life and work, everything will get done and we will all feel more fulfilled in our work. You know how it feels to go to work at a job when your heart is not in it. We've all been there. Really, then it is just a job. And guess what? Your clients feel it too. If you are not so thrilled to be at work, it comes through even when you think it doesn't. Conversely, when you enjoy your work because you feel a connection to your clients, they feel that too. They feel welcome because you are glad to see them. They feel attended to because you understand what they are feeling. Proverbs 29:18 says "Where there is no vision, the people perish." Vision is like walking into the candy store of life with a million dollar gift card. Pick what you like! Look around and dare to believe you can have what you want by deciding first what it IS that you want, and then diligently go about creating it.

34

Never having been an athlete as a child, I was an adult before I learned that being involved in sports teaches people valuable lessons about success. One of those lessons involves vision. Athletes are commonly taught to look where they want to go. In the literal sense, keeping your head up to look where you want to go, rather than looking down at where you are, will help get you to where you want to be. Make this a habit by starting every day with your list of goals in front of you. Ask yourself which goals you will work on by doing the tasks you can do today. Pretty soon this exercise will become second nature. When you have a slow day or week, it won't get you down because you will already be in the habit of doing what you are able. The extra time you have will improve your situation/practice/skills. In the words of legendary coach John Wooden, "Do not let what you *cannot* do interfere with what you can do."

When you enjoy your work, it shows in everything you do. Choose your preferred population and go for it. Find ways to market yourself to that population through volunteer work or donations or specials. Word will get around when someone from your target market comes to you and loves your work. My pet project is teachers. I feel teachers have the second hardest job in the world right behind parents, and sometimes the teachers have to act like parents, too. Therefore, I chose teacher appreciation events for my volunteer work early on, and I go to a few schools every year and donate time to giving chair massage to all the teachers who want to participate. Although I planned for this to be a form of my giving back, from the very first event I got a client who I saw monthly for years thereafter, and she brought me three more clients. I gave, and I received much more. Teachers fall into that overworked person category, a population of caring people who are always putting the needs of others first, and sometimes they need a little convincing to take some time for themselves.

Pay attention to the details

Keep excellent notes on what your individual clients like. Is her favorite part of massage when you rub her feet? Her scalp? His back? Clients have their own preferences on heat and will appreciate you greatly if you keep them warm, or conversely keep the heat low because they tend to get hot. Does your client have arthritis in her hands? Always use warm mitts to soothe her hands and she will be grateful to you for your extra attention. It is especially important for male therapists to understand what women want because sometimes the comforts to women are hard for a man to imagine. Some men seldom get cold, but women get cold much more quickly so it's important to keep them warm. Also, pay special attention if you have a client who you know is prone to have hot flashes. These are the details that will help you stand out from the crowd and keep your clients comfortable and remembering YOU! You are demonstrating how much you care by paying attention to these details.

Professionalism, Integrity, and Character

Once you get a new client, you certainly will want them to come back. Some people will come back because they like your massage techniques. Others will stay with you because they feel more comfortable with you than with other therapists they have tried. Perhaps your location is the top motivating priority, or it could be your price is right for their budget. Underneath all these reasons, however, is who you are and how you make the client feel. Who you are, how you present yourself, and your presence in telephone conversations or in-person conversations, all give the other person the chance to observe your professionalism, integrity, and character. Remember, every person you meet everywhere is a potential client. These are by far your most valuable marketing tools for yourself and your practice. If you are a peaceful, positive, and caring person and you exhibit those behaviors everywhere you are, people will be drawn to you. Colleagues, fellow parishioners, neighbors, even friends and family will be more likely to feel comfortable coming to you for massage therapy. On the other hand, if you are often seen acting in an unfeeling way toward others, and then you switch over to your professional mode when it's work time, it may be too late. An impression has already been formed in the mind of the other person. There is a Buddhist saying, "The way you do one thing is the way you do everything."

Here is an example of an excellent way to demonstrate your integrity and character. You will often receive calls from people who start the conversation by saying they are looking for a massage therapist. Often they will ask first about your fees. They may give you details of the discomfort they are experiencing. You might even offer advice of things they can do at home to help such as specific stretching exercises or applying heat or ice. They may even ask about your availability. In the end, they may or may not book an appointment. Rather than feel frustrated that you gave your time and talents without them booking an appointment, be glad they called you and gave you the opportunity to talk. They may be looking for a quick and free fix, but more often they are truly not ready to book an appointment for whatever reason. The advice you give will show them that you honestly care more for their health than your bottom line. Your focus on serving will be evident and appreciated. You may be surprised to find the same person calling again a few weeks or even months later, ready to book the appointment and pay you for your time. Your generosity in talking with them may have been just what they needed to feel comfortable with you. Now is your chance to show what you can do once you have them on your table. Sowing seeds of warm professionalism and helpfulness will always pay off one way or another.

Maturity and Long-Term Focus

Long term success requires long term focus and maturity. Maturity is knowing that we need to string together a lot of successful weeks and months to survive in business for the long run. Too often new therapists who legitimately need an income immediately will give their practice three months or six months to pay off or they quit. Maturity says I'm focusing on my goal of five massages per week for the first six months and doing everything I can to make that happen. Maturity says I can adjust my goal higher once I start reaching my initial goal some of the time. Progress is being made with each successful massage you give. Be patient. Stay focused on your progress and your goals. The clients will come. The profits will increase. As more clients come to you, like your style, and talk with their friends and neighbors about the great massage they got from you (referrals!), the more your phone will ring and your days will begin to fill up. You build momentum once you get these numbers moving, and the numbers take on a life of their own. More people talking about the great massage you gave them leads to more calls and more clients and so on!

One very easy way to impress new clients in the early months is to be absolutely sure you have a clean office, smooth sheets, a quiet atmosphere, and a safe environment. These are the basics that will build trust for you and build rapport with you. Put yourself in your client's shoes and stand in your doorway and pretend you are looking into the office of another professional, not your own office. What do you see? Is the waiting area tidy, warm, inviting, and quiet? Is your treatment room secure? Are the blinds or curtains closed? Are the table linens smooth or do they look like they have been pulled from the laundry basket where they obviously spent the last few days? Is the room properly lit for a client to feel comfortable? Is the temperature right? Keep in mind that the client's initial reaction of feeling welcome or uneasy will carry over into the massage. You haven't even touched the client yet, but the first impression they get of you from your office space will set the tone for the massage itself. (We will get more into the details of what physical excellence looks like in the next section.) When the client can see you have taken the time to set up an excellent space, he or she will begin to relax.

Once I saw a new client in my early months and I did everything I could think of to help him feel comfortable by showing him that I was strictly professional. Still, when I came back into the room after he had time to undress and get on the table, I immediately noticed that he had carefully placed his shoes right by the door, side by side and pointing out. Wow, here is someone who, just in case, is ready to run if necessary. I was glad I noticed the shoes because it told me I needed to be absolutely sure I did all I could to help him feel comfortable and see that he could trust me. I kept the conversation geared to my pressure, his response to my pressure, and explained each technique as I progressed from working on his neck and shoulders to arms and so on. I listened to him breathe and heard his breathing slow and become deeper as time went on. Eventually, he even went to sleep. Success! I did everything I could to show this client he could trust me, and it worked.

Listening is very important

Show every client you are listening. Give the client in your office your full attention. Do more listening than talking. Listen twice as much as you talk. Ask lots of pertinent questions regarding your pressure and their comfort. The client will tell you what they want to solve that day and in the long term if you ask. They will tell you what they like about massage. They will tell you about negative experiences in previous massages and you will know precisely what not to do! If you are listening, you will learn how to serve them well. If they feel listened to, they will see that you care. Clarify anything you are not sure you understand. Exactly where in the back are they feeling this discomfort, and during what actions? You will be helping the client relax and know you are fully present. They will realize they are more likely to get a good massage for their money and time. After all, they can go elsewhere for massage therapy. Remember that always. Give them reasons to want to come back to you. And when this client has a good experience by feeling that you truly care, he or she is likely to talk about it with someone else too.

When your client is on the table and mentions a hobby or an interest, it is natural to want to say so if you share that hobby or interest. Stay curious about your client, however. Be sure to toss the conversation right back to the client. I find it helpful in creating connections with clients to talk about any common interests while keeping in mind that their massage time is truly their time. I let them decide whether or not we will have a chat about our shared interest, or how long that chat will go. If I realize I'm doing most of the talking and they have become quiet, we have lost our balance and I may be infringing on the client's time.

With new clients, I usually even tell the person right up front that this time is theirs alone, and they get to decide if they prefer to talk or have quiet. Many people in our society feel uncomfortable with silence, or feel they are being rude if they let a conversation drag or stall. I want them to know they are not here to entertain me. Then I do my best to stick to it!

Devoting time to your practice

Devote a set amount of time each week to your practice. Decide the amount of time that is right for you by considering if you eventually want to be full time or part time, and whether or not you are still working at another part-time job. When you find yourself with no appointments for an afternoon, go to the office anyway for an hour or two and study your anatomy book. I can't tell you how many times I did this in the early months, and while I was up to my mastoid processes in refreshing my memory of muscle groups and boney landmarks, the phone rang. A prospective client called to check on my prices and availability. Because I didn't take the afternoon off to go shopping, I was able to look at the clock and calculate a reasonable time to offer, saying "I happen to have an opening at 3:30 today, or I have time tomorrow too". The person on the other end of the phone does not need to know you have been open all afternoon. More often than not, you have just made the prospective client's day because often the person calling has time available when they call and are delighted that you are offering time today or tomorrow. Dedicating a pre-determined amount of time to be in your work space always pays off one way or another. Often it results in more clients because you were available to answer the phone and promote yourself in a professional manner without the caller hearing in the background "Clean-up in aisle 6!" If a caller hears that, what will he think? Hmmm, is she a full time professional therapist or part time? Now there is nothing wrong with working part time if that is your goal and you are completely up front with it. But if you plan to make massage your career and you want to make a good living at it, being available within your predetermined hours and days will really pay off. That availability will draw in callers and clients. The universe knows what you need and where your heart is focused. If you are still working at another job early on and you need to keep that income for a while, certainly make that part of your weekly schedule, but set up a reasonable amount of time to devote to your practice and stick to it whether your appointments are filled or not.

When I started massage school, I went to work in a bakery as a cake decorator. Once I passed my boards and could receive payment for massage, it didn't take too many massages per week to match and surpass the income I had been earning. I resisted the urge to work both jobs for a while, knowing if I was not obligated to be in the bakery, then I would be more available when clients called for an appointment. My focus was solely on building a successful private practice. I cut out every expense possible so I could do without the extra job in order to keep myself available every day. Can you cut your expenses anywhere? Look again! Can you cut back on eating in restaurants and save money there? Which would you rather have, another client who could turn into a regular client or someone to cook a meal for you? Can you make coffee at home or watch that movie on DVD instead of in the theater? Wear the clothing you have longer? Cutting expenses wherever possible might free up enough money in your budget to quit that part time job and focus on your massage therapy practice.

Honestly, even with cutting expenses everywhere possible you might still need to work your other job a few days each week. I'm not suggesting you go broke waiting for your phone to ring. Keep that part time job as long as you need to, but structure your work time around it and around your other obligations so that you are in the office sometimes even when you don't have an appointment scheduled. Set up your schedule around the hours you want to work. Devote your time to preparing yourself for the success you desire. Focus, focus, focus! Eat, sleep, and breathe massage therapy in the early months. You will be building a strong foundation for your practice and you will succeed!

Remember that once you get the ball rolling, momentum will keep the ball moving. You will have all the important early decisions made and habits of excellence in place in every part of your work. Soon you will be able to relax and enjoy more free time. Henry David Thoreau said it quite well: "If one advances confidently in the direction of his dreams, and endeavors to live the life which he has imagined, he will meet with success unexpected in common hours." It's true! You can do this!

Building your own physical strength

Build your strength slowly and steadily early on. In the beginning, five massages per week is an excellent number for several reasons. Massage therapy is very physical. It takes time to build the muscles you will eventually need to work on three, four, five, or more people every day. Starting out with a "full" schedule, whatever that means to you, is not a healthy way to start your practice. You will invite injury and find yourself on the disabled list before long. Then watch the income drop like a lead balloon. But what to do with all that time that seems to be free time? First, see the list above. It's not free time, it's investment time! You are investing in your practice, your health, and your clients' health. Second, make exercise and stretching a priority to help build your strength and keep your muscles flexible. If you have not already been following a fitness routine, now is the time to start. No ifs, ands, or buts. Being a massage therapist is physical and demanding, so you need to take care of yourself. You will feel better, you will feel more confident in your abilities, and you will be more likely to think clearly. Also, you will be a healthy health-care provider, and that speaks well for your professionalism. You need to be practicing healthy activities while helping your clients be healthy too. People pay attention to whether or not you live and follow your own advice. Don't just talk the talk, but also walk the walk, as they say.

The difference between a successful person and others is not a lack of strength, not a lack of knowledge, but rather a lack of will.

Vince Lombardi

Where are your thoughts?

Okay, let's take a fork in the road here. What are you thinking right now? Why? These are important questions for you to ask yourself. Be honest about your answers. Are you thinking "I will never get this, what was I thinking?" Or are you thinking "I am a massage therapist. This is a bit scary, but exciting! I can do this!" Long ago I cut a quote from the newspaper and have had it posted on my refrigerator ever since. You may be familiar with it:

Be careful of your thoughts, for your thoughts become your words. Be careful of your words, for your words become your actions. Be careful of your actions, for your actions become your habits. Be careful of your habits, for your habits become your character. Be careful of your character, for your character becomes your destiny.

The author was listed as unknown, but I think the message is priceless and timeless. Pay close attention to what you think about during a massage and outside the massage room too. If energy follows attention, and I believe it does, paying attention to your thoughts really pays off. I went to a therapist who seemed to be angry. Her techniques were appropriate but her touch was too rough. As we chatted I learned that she was going through a rough period in her life. I went back a few times to see if perhaps that first day was just a bad day. Well, it seemed to be a prevailing attitude. Although she knew how to massage well, I could feel her anger and no matter how many times I asked her to ease up on the pressure, she continued on with the rough treatment while she talked about her problems. I know she was technically a good therapist, but whatever thoughts were swirling through her head as she told me about this or that injustice in her life were coming through her hands. No thanks.

Although some people are more sensitive to feeling energy than others, I assume that all my clients can feel my energy to some degree and I want to make sure they feel positive energy! Also, focusing on how tight a muscle is can be counterproductive. Instead, when I find a tight area the words in my head are "release, ease, health". I want my attention to be on healing, so energy goes to **healing**. I want my clients to feel good about their massage appointment today because they feel comfortable and welcome and cared for. How can I help them feel comfortable when I am uncomfortable? Impatient? Cranky? Sure we all have moods, but paying attention to what we are thinking and feeling will help us attend to the client in front of us and express compassion, peace, and kindness.

When I find myself feeling cranky or tired during my workday, I take a few minutes to use a grounding exercise to balance my energy and tune into positive energy around me. If you are not already using a grounding exercise, try mine. I think about my feet being firmly planted on the ground. All negative energy can exit my body through my feet and go into the ground where it can be recycled into positive energy. I think about the top of my head being connected to the higher power and positive energy, inviting it to fill me with light, healing energy, and love. This practice always helps me to let go of any negative feelings or thoughts and be centered again where I can be fully present to my clients.

Do your best to honor your clients by giving them your full attention. They are paying you for an hour of your time and that means more than just your hands. Don't disconnect your hands from your brain and heart by tuning out and going off into space with thoughts of what to have for lunch. Don't spend your energy wondering if you left the window open at home or whether or not you have enough clients on the calendar next week while your hands are going through the motions of massage. The person on the table WILL KNOW if you are fully there or not. Your thoughts show up in everything you do whether you realize it or not. Stay focused on what you feel in their muscles and keep your intention toward healing. Listen to what they say. Listen to how they breathe. Listen to your intuition.

We all get distracted at times, and I am no exception! Therefore, I adopted a mantra that I use to guide me back to the room when I find that I have drifted away. As soon as I realize I am thinking outside the massage room instead of focusing on the person I'm working on, I switch my thoughts to 'health and well-being'. I use these four words as a mantra, repeating them over and over again to re-focus all of my attention. This is my prayer for the person on whom I'm working, and now I am back in the room where I need to be, focusing on the muscles I feel and determining how much pressure and time they need. Your client will definitely feel the difference and relax knowing she is in good hands (pun intended).

Relax and be yourself

Of course you can do everything "right" and still have people who do not come back to you. It happens to everyone. Sometimes it is a personality difference, sometimes it's your style, and maybe it is just not a good fit. It could be as simple as your location. Personality can play a big role in building your business and your best strategy is to just be you. You cannot be everything to everyone, so relax and be yourself. You will build trust as clients recognize the connection you have made with them and the two of you will build rapport. On the other hand, some clients won't connect with you. That doesn't mean you are doing something wrong. It might just mean the two of you have different styles, and that's okay. It is important for you to develop your own style knowing that your style will not fit everyone.

I have learned a tremendous amount by visiting a lot of therapists over the years and I have seen a wide variety of contrasting approaches. For instance, I like to keep my table soft and warm. I went to a therapist using minimal cushioning on the table under the sheets, and no warmer. It turns out the preferred type of client in this practice is someone dealing with an injury, coming in weekly for work that is targeted on that particular part. Clothing is not removed, and little or no work is done on any other part of the body. Therefore, they do not need the cushioning and warmth I prefer to use. Even though I am often working to resolve uncomfortable neck or back issues for clients, I also want to keep them warm, give a full body massage if appropriate, and help them relax completely to encourage whole-body healing.

Conversely, a therapist who plays loud or heavy music is also interested in attracting a different type of client than I am. That is great too. There are plenty of styles of therapist and plenty of different clients. Once you know your preferred style, set up your practice the way you want it. Build rapport with each new client coming to you by being the best YOU!

Sometimes people would come to me for a first visit and when it came time to talk about their preferences on pressure, they would literally use the words "beat me up", saying no amount of pressure was too much. I didn't know how to handle that at first, and I gave them the firm pressure I felt was appropriate for the muscles I worked on. Sometimes they liked the massage and came back, and sometimes not. With time, experience, and confidence I started speaking up for myself, answering their request by telling them up front that I have a gentle style. Gentle did not mean I could not or would not be effective at getting into the appropriate muscle depth and relieve the client's discomfort or restriction. Gentle means everything I do is with kindness and respect, focus and intention. By proceeding gently I always know what I am feeling and don't take chances on causing harm to the client or to myself. More than once a client who had asked for deep pressure came out of the room saying he didn't think he would feel much affect from the massage but he was wrong. He said he felt completely different when he got up.

Who doesn't like to be treated with kindness? How do you feel when you are treated with kindness? How do you feel when you are treated with indifference or disrespect? How do you want your clients to feel?

Then again if the client asked you three times during the massage to use more (or less) pressure or less heat, maybe this person isn't going to turn into a long term client, and that's okay. One therapist I visited began my massage with a scalp rub, which is normally my favorite spot. However, his pressure was so intense I had to tell him immediately that he needed to lighten up a lot. His response was "Really? I figured I'd give you my athlete's massage since you are so athletic." It doesn't matter what you call it, one size does not fit all. He listened to me and lightened up, but I had to remind him several times through the massage to lighten up again, and I got a good massage. Clearly though, I was not his ideal client nor was he my ideal therapist. That's okay. There are plenty of clients who need and want that kind of intense pressure and I was happy to direct them to him! His heart was in the right place and he was a good therapist, just not for me.

Quite often people would come to me saying the last therapist they saw caused bruising and did not back off when asked to reduce the pressure. Remember that no matter how effective you feel you are, if the client is in pain because of your pressure and leaves your office feeling roughed up, they are not going to be happy. How likely are they to come back? Long ago before I ever thought about becoming a massage therapist, I was on a massage table when the therapist found a knot in the middle of my back. I had been taking piano lessons and developed a strain there, so I knew she had found a good spot that needed to be worked on. However, she focused on that one spot for so long and used so much pressure that I was barely able to breathe. I didn't know at the time that I could ask her to lighten up! I figured she knew what she was doing. I knew the spot was there. When I got to the point where I felt I had endured enough pain in that spot and was beginning to tell her that's enough, she moved on, and I could breathe again. The rest of the massage was comfortable. It was just that one spot where she had stayed and focused that I was not comfortable. After the massage,

49

though, for three full days I could not move in any way without significant pain full across my back. Needless to say, I was not a happy client. Interestingly enough though, after three days the spot and the pain were both gone completely and did not come back, so yes the therapy was effective. I was thankful for that, but I knew there had to be a better way because the price I paid in true pain was far too high at the time of the massage and for the three days afterward. I compare this type of work to a teenager having braces to straighten teeth. How many parents would provide this beneficial treatment for their kids if the orthodontists tried to achieve full straightening in one month?

One client I worked on even said his wife would be very glad he got a massage from me. I asked why. He said she loves getting massages from him but she is always asking him to lighten up with the pressure. He said he thought she was being a wimp and he was doing what he felt she needed. He was amazed to receive a gentle but effective massage. He could not wait to try it on her. That is my style and I am sticking to it. I know myself, my strengths, my preferences, and I want to enjoy my work, not dread it. Be kind to your clients, always. And be kind to yourself.

No matter how hard we try, **we will not please everyone**! That's okay. Massage therapists have different styles and so do clients. There are enough clients for all of us so stick with your style and be happy every day doing work you love without over extending your time, strength, or interests.

By understanding this concept of differing styles and expectations, you can honor each client by suggesting an alternate therapist whose style better matches this client's preferences. Now you have made them happy by validating their preferences and giving them guidance in finding the right therapist for them. Now that they recognize your kindness, they will be more likely to refer someone they know who is looking for a therapist with your style. What goes around comes around.

Understanding what people want

Remember the movie from long ago with Mel Gibson called *What Women Want*? Gibson's character suddenly could read the minds of women around him and he learned a great deal. We cannot actually read minds, but we can understand some basic principles that bring clients to see us.

As you know, people come in for massage for a variety of reasons. Everyone comes from their own point in life's journey, and none of us knows exactly what path others are on. Most people are coming for massage therapy first and foremost. But after that, or in addition, some people crave human interaction and/or the touch of another human being. Do they live alone? Is their family all scattered around the country?

Others need a sounding board for ideas floating through their head or for some pressing decision. Some want to check out of their busy week and get away from it all on your massage table where they can dream and rest while having tension worked out of their muscles. And then some may get massage to solve that issue that has been stumping them all week, knowing once they get on the table and forget about the outside world the right answer will suddenly appear.

Remember that the client is a whole person, not just a set of muscles to be worked. Listen to them. Learn what you need to know to help them relax and feel better. Honor them exactly where they are, without any judgment. No labels are needed. If you get a client who lives with constant pain and seems to go on about how bad they feel, resist the urge to call them a whiner, even in your own thoughts. Some people handle pain more quietly than others. Some need to talk about it, to be heard. Either way, each person is doing the best they can. Whether or not you understand a client's motives for coming in for massage therapy, you can affirm:

- I give people the beautiful feeling of well-being.
- I relieve pain from people's bodies.

- I regularly help people create breakthroughs in the cycle of pain.
- I regularly help people feel better than they thought possible.
- I regularly help people relieve pain they previously thought they'd have to learn to live with forever.

Keeping your thoughts in the positive realm will help you to help them have a better day regardless of the reason they have come to see you. In a workshop once I witnessed a fellow therapist ask the presenter what to do if you just don't like the client. Great question! And the presenter's answer was even better: **Treat everyone with unconditional positive regard**. Right on. I was glad to hear that and remembered it ever since. Everyone deserves unconditional positive regard. You and the client will both have a better day.

You will sometimes see clients who have an injury or an ache that needs attention and once it is gone they won't be back until the next time it flares up. Others know the value of regular massage for maintaining health throughout life and they will make their next appointment with you as they pay for today's session. Let each person guide you in their preferences and refer anyone who prefers a style that is just not you. Don't waste time or energy feeling bad that you didn't have a good match. Embrace your uniqueness and respect each client. Be yourself and enjoy your work! Don't ever try to be something or someone you are not, and you and your clients will be happier! Clients meant for you will find you, I promise!

Honor each client

Another way to honor each client is to watch for subtle signs of discomfort. In general, most people will not speak up if they are mildly uncomfortable. I've done it, and you probably have too! What are we thinking? When I'm the one on the table, I'm thinking, hmmm, do I seem to need that particular spot worked on this long? I like to give the therapist the benefit of the doubt. Or maybe I am tired that day and don't want to go to the effort to speak up. Sometimes the client is too shy to say anything. Once when I asked a client if the pressure I was using was okay, she responded by asking me if she had a choice! Of course she has the final word on pressure. Be the therapist who honors the client by giving them the proper pressure. Sometimes they don't want to complain! My thought is that clients are not complaining when they are telling of their discomfort to a person who can do something about it. So if they don't speak up, watch for body language to be your best guide. Some common signs of discomfort are wincing, shallow breathing, or slightly pulling the arm or leg away from you. Learn to pay attention to each client and pick up on their way of communicating with you. They will appreciate you all the more for it. Dave Foster said it well in his book *Accept No Mediocre Life* when referring to your personal investment in your own excellence: "The road is long and hard, but it's not crowded and the rewards are limitless."

Professional Boundaries

Set appropriate boundaries right from the start or as early as possible if you are already practicing. It's much harder – but still possible – to impose boundaries later on. Once you have let clients develop a habit of calling you at the last minute to change an appointment, it is hard to say no. We do our best to be available but there is a limit to appropriate flexibility. We do not want to give our clients the impression they can either expect us to be available to them at any moment or expect to cancel late and leave us hanging. Once you decide what your cancellation policy will be, print it out and display it prominently in your office. Include it on your web site. Be sure it is clearly stated in your brochure that you give each new client.

When I was new I had a client who wanted to book a standing appointment every Wednesday night for two hours. I was open to the time slot for a few weeks but I knew this could not be permanent. I also could not quite believe this would be a regular thing! Once I saw that he really meant he would come back every week, I tried to persuade him to pick another evening. I hope I did a good job when I told him I appreciated the opportunity to work with him but Wednesday evening is the night for choir practice, and I could not and would not miss practice on a regular basis. I told him we would need to find another time or day, and he did not come back. Literally, he was asking me to make a choice, and as much as I wanted regular clients, I was not willing to give up something that was very important to me. I have never forgotten that situation and choice I made, and I have never regretted it. I would have loved to continue to book that client regularly, but he was adamant about the day and time. So was I. I took care of myself and kept my own priorities in mind. If I had no other obligations on that particular evening, that would have been a totally different situation. Find a way to say kindly what you will do and what needs to be adjusted.

Another common boundary issue is family members who want us to work on them when we get together for social events. Give this point some thought ahead of the next event so you can be ready. Do you want to always be giving Uncle Steve twenty free minutes of treatment at family gatherings? Go ahead if you want to. You might very well have a good reason to do it. If not, however, the next time you are going to see him at a birthday dinner, be ready with your schedule and tell him kindly that you are off duty tonight but you would love to work out that kink in his neck. How would Thursday evening at 7:00 be? You are being professional and direct. This also sends a message to the rest of the family. You are serious about your new profession and you keep regular business hours. Your free time is just that – your time.

When family members do want to make appointments, decide what your payment policy will be up front. I have too big a family to give massage away free, so I decided I was comfortable with half price. That way I am giving them a special rate but I do not feel I am being used. Also, they do not have to hesitate to call me, wondering if they are taking advantage of me. I am being compensated and I am happy to reduce the rate for my special peeps. Remember, you do not have to do it the way I did it. The point is, decide early what you want to do and state it clearly and kindly when needed. You do not want to start dreading going to family events because you find yourself working half the evening. Or maybe you do. Just give it some serious thought so you can be ready and show respect for yourself and your family.

Suppose some time has gone by and you find yourself with a client who has gotten into the habit of calling you at the last minute to change his appointment. As hard as it feels, it is actually easier to speak up than to go on feeling frustrated and losing business. Tell him that as much as you want to accommodate his schedule changes, you are busy enough now that you don't have too many other openings. Tell him that you need to be sure that he will be there for the time you have reserved for him. You are not being disrespectful of him as a client. You are showing respect for yourself, your practice as a whole, and exhibiting your professionalism. No doctor's office would allow repeat last-minute changes like that without appropriate consequences. They have cancellation policies too.

Then there are the clients who always seem to call on the day you are busiest and ask for an appointment that same day. While it is great to have open time in the early months and be able to see someone the same day, the time will come when you need more notice to schedule an appointment. Most people understand this completely. What happens, though, to all of us sooner or later, is that we will have a client with a hectic schedule who is not able to plan even a week in advance. With these folks, I apologize when telling them I do not have any openings today and make sure I sound like I mean it! I tell them I understand their schedule will not allow for earlier planning, and we come to an agreement. They call whenever they want to and I tell them honestly if I have an opening or not. They know I will do everything I can to accommodate their schedule, but they appreciate knowing that I will be honest with them. They know I will not add them to the end of my day if they are not likely to get a good massage from me when I'm tired and/or frustrated! We both win because I have created a way for both of us to be served. Always aim for win-win.

Eliminating as many sources of frustration as possible allows for more peace for you, your clients, and throughout your whole practice.

Gratitude

Remember to do your best to keep an attitude of gratitude. Today is a great day for many reasons! What is your first thought when you wake up in the morning on a work day? Ugh, a feeling of tiredness, or even dread? However, what if you experience every work day morning having the same positive energy as the first day of vacation? You can if you inhabit a space of gratitude. Ah, what a day this will be!

I recommend saying "thank you" when you first wake up in the morning.   I say thank you for a good night's sleep. Thank you for this day. Thank you for this opportunity to work and make a living. Thank you that today will be a great day. Thank you for the clients who are coming to see me today. Thank you for meaningful work. Thank you for the blessings of serving and making a difference in the world. Thank you for indoor running hot water with which to shower and start my day! Thank you for an abundance of food, and refrigeration to keep it fresh. Thank you for my health which allows me to work.

Now, what do you think would happen if you made a practice of saying every morning: today is a great day because...then fill in the blank. Today is a great day because my workload is lighter than usual! Today is a great day because I have a full day! Today is a great day because I have no meetings! Today is a great day because I'm finally going to start that project I've been procrastinating on. Because I'm going to finish that project I've been working on for weeks. Because I lost another pound. Because I'm seeing two of my most upbeat clients today. Because several of my clients have been showing great progress in their health and they believe in massage. Because, because, because. There are so many reasons today is a great day. It's going to rain and we need it. The sun is coming back out and we've missed it. My roses are blooming. My grandson smiled for the first time!

As you go on with your day, keeping any positive thoughts will help you notice other details that make it a great day. Positive things are everywhere and just waiting to be noticed. And do you know what? Your clients will feel your happiness. You will feel more confident. You will enjoy your day more. You will have more strength. At the end of the day you will be wondering why this day seemed so easy. It's not really a mystery. Your attitude makes all the difference, and your clients are directly affected. How you feel shows up on your face, in your hands, and in how you carry yourself.

Here's another great trick: when I look at my schedule for the next day or week and I see that I have two clients tomorrow or seven clients for the week, I always add the words 'so far'. I have two clients tomorrow, so far. I have seven clients this week, so far. I am intentionally opening my mind and my schedule to increase and abundance. I am inviting more clients to call and book appointments. Adding those two words has increased my prosperity many times.

The fact that you notice the reasons for the great day doesn't mean the challenges and less-than-pleasant aspects of a day do not exist. They are still there, but they will not have the same power over you when you give your time and attention and energy toward changing the challenges into positives. Negatives drain us, and positives empower us. Use this phenomenon to your advantage. Not sure it will work? Just for today, try it. Don't worry if a few negatives creep into your awareness. Acknowledge them and move on to the next task and the next reason to be happy. Tomorrow, try again. And again the next day. Do it for three weeks and make it a habit. Watch your health flourish, and watch your clients respond. Watch your phone ring and your practice grow.

Honestly, I start most days this way, and I guarantee when I do start this way, the day goes much better! I continue this attitude of gratitude throughout the day and through each massage, thanking God for blessing each client with healing energy, peace, and love. At the end of the day I say thank you as I turn off each light, the music, the warmers, everything. Fill your day, your work, your mind, and your heart with gratitude. Watch the blessings pour in.

Keep a Journal

I recommend that you keep a daily log or journal at least your first year, but two to three years would be even better because it takes a while to build a full practice. The industry average is four to five years. You will learn something new each and every day. School is only part of the training. Now you are in the real 'wonderful world of massage' as I call it, and it can be discouraging to find out how much you still need to learn. Don't let it get you down. It is the same in any job, any profession. The bigger the learning curve, the more challenging – and rewarding – the field. Write down any observations you have made, techniques you feel more confident with, changes to your medical history process, and even the number of clients you are seeing in a week and how you feel about all of it. On a slow day or week, take the time to go back and read some early entries. You will soon realize you have made some real and excellent progress in your feelings of competence and confidence. And let's face it, massage therapy is a confidence game. Confidence is everything, and once you realize you can do this, you will work with greater ease, less doubt, and the success will snowball!

Trading Massages

If you are lucky enough to be in a situation where you trade massages with colleagues, do not make the mistake of thinking these are free massages. Not only do you pay for the massage you get with your time – and how much is that worth? – but these are also valuable networking opportunities. Treat trading opportunities and therapists with all the respect you feel toward your clients paying with money. In the early years of my practice I made notes on every massage I gave and received in trade. I learned more techniques, practiced being professional, and gained physical strength with each massage I gave. Every time a colleague gives you the opportunity to work on them, they deserve at least all the same respect, if not more than, a paying client. They actually are paying you in experience. Do not cancel them at the last minute unless you absolutely have to. Give them your full attention. Treating them like the paying client they actually are will show them you are a true professional. In addition to all the benefits already mentioned, you never know when they may call on you to work with them on a chair massage event that requires more than one therapist. Also, they might start referring clients to you when they are not available. If you treat them with less than full professionalism, how likely are they to call you when they need the assistance of another professional?

Be Confident

Do some clients intimidate you? Why? Give that some thought. We all have times when we feel less than adequate, and being a new therapist is full of those times. We are asking people to come to us for treatment and frankly that is scary! Just out of school, unless you've worked on a lot of extra practice clients, it takes time to build enough experience that allows us a level of comfort in feeling prepared regardless of what conditions our new clients present to us. Do not let fear take over.

It is inevitable that you will feel some fear. I felt plenty! I was afraid of everything in the beginning! But fear sucks the life out of every idea, every dream, every goal if we are not careful. Being courageous is not the absence of fear, it is forging ahead in spite of fear.

To help you feel more confident in the beginning, remember that as a human being while you are not better than anyone else, it is also true that no one else is better than you. I was comfortable with the first thought in that sentence for decades before I got the second part into my head and heart. Wow, what a difference that made. I knew I was not better than anyone else, but deep down I really did believe everyone was better than me. Once I realized my error, I KNEW I could succeed because I did not need to be intimidated by any clients or any situation.

Replace any and all doubt or worry with positive statements. Tell yourself daily "I will succeed!" Fear has been called False Events Appearing Real. Quite often fear is a result of misinterpretation of a situation. Have you noticed that most of the things we fear never come to pass? If you are on equal ground as everyone you work on, what is there to fear? Believe in yourself! Trust in your abilities! Believe that you are right where you are meant to be and want to be. Act with courage. Remember, too, that you are never alone. With God, all things are possible. Proceed with confidence and know that you are able to work and live in peace and love, not fear.

While you are building your confidence, take a load of pressure off yourself by remembering that you can not fix everything. I used to have the attitude that I needed to fix everything, but I did not even realize it. A classmate in massage school pointed it out to me. What a relief I felt when I realized it is not my responsibility to fix the world! That was a huge weight off my shoulders. Certainly we all want to do what we can to make life around us as pleasant as possible. That is a far cry, though, from trying to fix everything and feeling the pressure of being responsible.

Becoming a massage therapist will automatically make you feel inadequate when someone doesn't feel great after their massage and achieve complete relief from their pain or discomfort. As wonderful as you are as a massage therapist, with all your training and practice sessions, all your diligence in learning techniques so you can make everyone feel better, all your focus on your client, it will happen that someone will soon express a continuing feeling of discomfort at the end of your massage. We can not guarantee 100% results any more than doctors can. What we can be sure of, however, is being fully present to each client, intending to do everything we know how to promote healing, believe in the power of divine healing energy, and letting go of the results. Often times the client has been feeling the ache or pain creeping up for weeks or months before coming to you. It stands to reason that ailments that have been weeks, months, or even years in the making will not be relieved in one session. Do your best and look for progress. Do they feel better? Perhaps three to five sessions will be required before they start feeling significantly better. That is not your fault. It's not that you did something wrong or did not do something right. Is it realistic to expect that one hour of massage every week will balance out forty to sixty hours of sitting at a computer? Massage will help greatly, but the client also needs to stretch and move daily-this is life and reality.

We also cannot make the client come back when we know massage therapy is likely to resolve their muscle issue. Each client has the right to make his or her own decisions on what course of treatment feels right, what their budget will allow, and pursue that course. Give them time. They may come back, especially if they proceed down a medical path and their symptoms are not relieved quickly there either. Each person must find his or her way. Do what you are able, with confidence.

Being Peace

There is a difference between feeling peaceful and acting peaceful, and this is an area where you might have to fake it till you make it. Recently at a chair massage event at a local school, I marveled at the interaction between the teachers while they were visiting us for their 15 minutes of massage. It was clear to me which teachers felt comfortable in their own skin. Perhaps they were long-time teachers, working a long time in one school. Time certainly helps anyone feel comfortable and competent. It is the same in any profession. Experience helps us become comfortable as we gain confidence in our own competence. Until then, however, acting peaceful can help you get through the early times of doubt. Be comfortable knowing you are doing the best you can do right now. Remember that you have studied a lot for this role. You have likely done many hours of practice massage already, possibly even hundreds of hours. You are a massage therapist. You can do this! Acting peaceful will help you remain calm and able to think clearly. See yourself as a confident, caring, successful massage therapist and you will become one! Some deep conscious breaths can help us get to a more peaceful and comfortable place even when we are not feeling peaceful.

Take Care of Yourself

Take care of yourself by scheduling your appointments responsibly and reasonably for your needs. Set boundaries like we talked about earlier. Use policy to enforce your boundaries by posting your policies in your office and on your website, and set them out very clearly with new clients. Restate your policies occasionally in your newsletter. Get plenty of rest for yourself. You will be so much more able to focus on your clients when you are rested and you too have recently had a massage. Be sure to do your best to exercise regularly. Build and balance your upper body muscles by lifting weights. Stretch your core and lower body with aerobic exercise and yoga or pilates. As noted earlier, building your practice slowly and naturally allows you to build not only the skills you need but also the muscles and stamina you will need for a long career. Taking care of yourself is a form of showing yourself and the world that you believe you are worth caring for. And you are! You have certainly heard that you cannot give away something you don't already have. Taking care of yourself fills your gas tank so you can go far. It also sets a good example for your clients. They are more likely to listen to your advice – and take it – when they see you live the way you recommend. You are a walking advertisement for your practice.

Being Competitive (in a constructive way)

Are you the competitive type who loves to win? Are you driven and ambitious? Let these qualities motivate you, but don't fall into the trap of comparing yourself to anyone else in any way. Measure your progress by your own standards and goals. Compete with last month's number of massages and last quarter's income so you are competing with your own track record. That drive to succeed will serve you well because you already have a burning desire to win. Just don't waste time and energy comparing yourself to other therapists when it comes to the bottom line. Every person is on his or her own journey, and blessings will come to all of us when we remain peaceful, helpful, and focused on our own progress. Remember that your life is unfolding just as it is meant to. As long as you are doing all you can possibly do to increase your business, you can remain calm and confident, which will invite prospective clients to you. You'll enjoy your work so much more, and your inner spirit guides will do the rest.

Giving vs. Marketing

Earlier I mentioned that I donate time to teacher appreciation events because this is a population I feel needs all the support we can give them. Although sometimes I meet teachers who subsequently become clients, this is not my focus at an appreciation event. I see these events as opportunities to give back to the community. I do give out my business cards if someone asks for one, but I do not go to the event loaded with promotional materials. I save my brochures, etc. for events where my focus is on marketing my skills and my practice. While we certainly need to market ourselves in many ways in the early years, be sure to include an occasional event where your intention is purely to give back. What is the difference? The difference is intention and results.

With marketing, we intend to showcase our massage skills in order to increase our client base. If a marketing event results in two to three new clients, we tend to repeat that type of event. If we get no new clients from a marketing event, we certainly will try another tactic to produce the results we want-more paying clients. However, with giving, the intention is to share kindness and give to others with no expectations of a payback. If we get new clients from a giving event, terrific! However, once I decide on my giving events for the year, I go to them repeatedly as long as I feel my efforts are reaching their intended mark. If I feel the population appreciates my presence, and their day/week/month is made better because I took time out of my schedule to give to them, that is all I need. That is my payoff for giving.

Giving is an act of karma. You've heard the sayings, "what goes around, comes around", and "we reap what we sow". Here is where our actions speak much louder than words. Every time we give, we are sowing seeds of kindness and health. Every time we give to another person, the universe/God/higher power takes note and we are paid back in some positive way. I believe giving is an important part of any life, any job, any relationship. Keep giving separate from marketing in your plans, and make sure to do some of each.

Hang in there!

Despite the advertisements you may have seen or heard, rarely does anyone make a large income right out of massage school. This is not a get rich quick business. It takes time to build up a client list, and that is true with almost any new business. Be patient. Work hard. Do your best. Keep at it. Plan your spending well. Don't spend all the money you make in a good week. Learn to budget your income in order to cover the slower weeks that are bound to happen. You will be able to relax more and attend to your clients with your full attention rather than worrying about your finances.

The beginning months and/or years will naturally be harder because everything is new and you are doing so much work to get the ball rolling. Loving your work does not mean you won't have to work hard, or that you won't have frustrations. Hard work and frustrations are a part of every life. When you willingly serve others, however, and you are fulfilling your purpose in life, you will feel a sense of accomplishment and joy. Feeling that your work is meaningful is very satisfying.

Do your best. Go the extra mile. Do all you can, and God will do the rest. I believe this. I believe we have access to supernatural power if we are open to it. The healing that happens in my office does not come solely from me. It comes through me from the universal healing energy, and that energy is available to every one of us. Focus on becoming the best therapist you can be. Use extra time available to study, market, exercise, and meditate. God is the ultimate healer as the creator of all that is good. With God all things are possible. When my time on this earth comes to an end and I meet God face to face, I very much hope to hear Him say "Well done my good and faithful servant". Hanging in there, being persistent, and doing our best, is doing enough and being enough.

Growing and maturing require understanding the balance between God's part and your part. You can't do God's part, and He won't do yours. The choice to grow smarter and stronger is yours and yours alone. The commitment to excel and go the extra mile starts within you.

David Foster, *Accept No Mediocre Life*

Part Two

Excellence is in the Details

The quality of a person's life is in direct proportion to their commitment to excellence, regardless of their chosen field of endeavor.

Vince Lombardi

This section will focus on the "how" to infuse your practice with excellence now that you have read about the "why". These ideas will help you keep your focus on creating excellence every day in every way possible for yourself and your clients. When your clients see and feel excellence in everything you do, they are likely to feel comfortable, feel welcome, and begin to trust you. I suggest reading this section all the way through at least once. Then you can go back and pick out a topic of interest one at a time as your focus for improvement today or this week. It makes me sad to hear about new therapists who quit after six months or a year of trying everything they know how to do. This world needs you! We need more health, more encouragers, and more peace. There is plenty of work for all of us so please stick with it until you find your own style and your own place in this wonderful business.

In the introduction section you read about how I got started – and why – in massage therapy. I talked about the fact that while I was a student I made up a schedule and signed up extra practice clients each week in order to be sure I had plenty of people on which to practice my lessons. The other benefit to giving away all those massages was to get people in the door to: 1) let them know I'm studying in a new field, and 2) to get them to try me or try massage. If you are in school, I implore you do to the same thing. Spread the word, make up a schedule, and start practicing like crazy! These are the benefits to you. As for the clients, everyone LOVES a bargain. People who know the value of massage will flock to you because they appreciate the opportunity to get massage free. Anyone who has not experienced a professional massage and is curious about it will be delighted at the chance to try it free. Look how many people you can make happy already!

If you are already practicing, I highly recommend you find ways to give away massage in an orderly fashion to get people in the door and give you a chance. Sure, it feels backwards to be giving away your time and talent – something that you just worked so hard to gain as your life's work. But giving away massages in the early days is priceless in gaining experience in working with a multitude of different people which leads to gaining confidence in yourself. I realize you need money now, but keep the long-term goal in mind. You just never know when the next weekly regular client might come along! Building a practice, whether you work for yourself or someone else, is a long process. Getting your name out there widely helps you immensely in building a following and building it faster. As more people come to you and then go out and talk about the fabulous massage they just got from you, the more new people will find you. I have sold quite a few gift certificates to a person I barely know who has never gotten a massage from me. But she knows people who have come to me, and they talk. This nice lady calls me when she needs a gift. And I so appreciate that!

Face it – you need the practice. Look at the other benefit to you. The pressure to do everything 'right' is greatly reduced because you know the person on your table understands that you are practicing to improve your skills. When you relax, more blood flows to your brain. You have more brain cells available to help you pay attention to what you are doing and feeling rather than worry about anything and everything.

Does that mean you can give less than 100%? Never! Treat every client, whether they have been with you for years or this is their first visit, free, self-paying, or using a gift certificate, as the one person who can make or break your practice. If you think that way every time a client walks through your door, such as 'this is the one I want to impress and work with for years', you will succeed! I once read that comedian Jerry Seinfeld started out doing two shows every night for eighteen months, no days off. All for free. He was not paid in dollars, but he was paid in practice opportunities and gained valuable experience. Look how it paid off for him. Now, let's get to the nitty-gritty details of how to make this happen for you!

Customer Service

Everything we are talking about could be considered customer service, but some points need to be made more specifically. Giving excellent customer service used to be the only way to be in business. The invention of voice mail and directive calling (press one for appointment, two for billing questions...) put a big dent in our ability to connect to our customers. Email is fantastic for silently leaving a message for someone at 3 am too. Technology is great with all the options we now have for contacting each other. However, nothing beats a real phone call for giving that important human touch.

If you receive an email requesting an appointment or massage information and the inquirer includes a phone number, I recommend sending them an email reply with all the information requested and then following up with a phone call. First, you have written down the information they requested and they can refer to it repeatedly as they wish. Second, when you call them you have far more opportunities to ask what the potential client is dealing with and engage them in a deeper conversation about how you can help with their stress or pain. Don't look at it as being pushy because you are merely assisting the client to make his or her day better. Again, we know how often we intend to accomplish the making of an appointment but it often gets put off. Calling the person who inquired about your services is a way of extending another service to them. Making that call, if you have their phone number, can often make the difference of resulting in an appointment or not. People love it when businesses are helpful.

Another way to show excellent customer service is by confirming your appointment with all new clients and for any appointment that was booked more than a week ago. Call them the day before their scheduled massage. It saves lost time for both you and the client. Everyone has the best

72

intentions but life happens. A person could get another call immediately after talking with you and forget to write down the information. You don't want to miss out on an opportunity to work, and the client really doesn't want to miss a scheduled massage. Then nobody is happy! Some therapists give reminder calls for every appointment. I started out that way, but almost everyone I called said they remembered and would be there, so I started calling only those I was not absolutely sure would remember their appointment. Again, we both win because they get their massage and we get the business.

Quality customer service builds trust and connection faster than anything else you do. Once you know the client will be there, make sure you are too! **Be on time for all appointments.** If your client is scheduled for 2:00, that means you need to do your best to arrive at least 30 minutes prior in order to have adequate time to turn on warmers, the music, review your notes, and clear your mind to be ready for this client. Being on time doesn't mean rushing in at a minute before 2:00! Of course there will be exceptions, as we all have been caught in unexpected traffic when an accident occurs. Your clients will be forgiving if it is an exception and you are normally in the office and ready for them when they arrive.

Show them you are serious about their comfort and well-being by making sure your workspace is as warm and inviting as it can possibly be. As noted earlier, stand in your doorway and pretend you are looking into the office of **someone else**. That will help you to be objective and really see what is before you. What feeling do you get? Is it inviting? Does the space appear professional? Is it **clean**? No matter how busy you are, take time for basics. Your office is another calling card – it says a lot about you and how much effort you put into your practice, which in turn says a lot about how much you care in general. Don't underestimate how important this is.

Look further: are the **pictures** on your walls calming, pleasing? Do you have items such as your policies and credentials posted that are informative? How about the overall feel of the space? Is it cozy or clinical? Both are fine. Just give it some thought so you achieve your personal goal. Wall decorations convey an atmosphere too. In my office I use a garden theme and many of my pictures contain flowers and birds. I also have taken the time to frame logos from professional organizations to which I belong, and some of the frames are garden-themed. Are your **rates** posted? Do you have a **cancellation policy** where clients can see it? Even better, you may want to make up an attractive page and put it in a nice frame saying "Quiet Zone. Please silence your cell phone".

Are your **linens** smooth and obviously clean and ready to put the client at ease? Really, I know we do a LOT of laundry, but folding the sheets promptly when they are dry will go a long way in building trust. If you walk into an office for a massage and you see linens that are very wrinkled, how do you know for sure they are clean? Give your clients peace of mind with smooth sheets!

Do you have a **mirror** placed where the client can check her appearance head to toe after the massage? For the first few years I had a small mirror on the wall at eye level. My eye level! Everyone is not 5'8", however. Once day I had a client come in who was a good foot shorter than me, and I realized my mirror was not at all helpful to her. I went out immediately and bought a full length mirror and hung it on the back of the treatment room door. Now she could see all of herself! All my clients would now be better served because they could check their whole appearance and feel properly put together when going on with their day. I felt really good about that change because I started to notice the mirror, or lack of it, when I visited other therapists. It's just plain helpful.

How about a large wall **calendar** in the area where clients normally conclude the visit with payment and thinking about the next visit? Many times the client trying to book their next appointment needed to look at my calendar to help them choose their next date. I did not want to show them my personal calendar for several reasons. It contains the names of other clients, and personal appointments as well. Putting up a wall calendar right where clients would be sitting or standing as they checked out was an excellent addition to the office. Again, very helpful! And calendars come in so many designs it is easy to find one that matches your décor and adds to the beauty and serenity of your space.

Is the **lighting** right for welcoming the client and allowing them to see that the space is clean and ready? You can turn off a lamp or two for ambience once the client is on the table, but be sure to turn on the lamp near their belongings before you leave the room so they can see to get dressed. I forgot to turn on the lamp near the client's chair once and when the client came out of the room she had turned on the obnoxious overhead lights! I never use those bright lights except to clean the office as they are far too harsh for massage. I felt awful that I had forgotten and vowed to remember to turn on the lamp for every client so they don't need to go for the overhead switch instead. In actuality the room is never completely dark as I have three small glowing-type lights that are always on during massage. It just happens that this client's need for light was greater than my own, and she taught me a valuable lesson by turning on the overhead lights.

Do you have a comfortable and sturdy place for the client to sit while **changing**? Sit in the chair and pretend you are the client. What does the client see from that chair? Is it pleasing and comforting? Is the space secure so the client knows he or she is not on display in any way? Does the chair have arms to assist any client who needs the extra help in getting up? Is the room **warm** enough for this client? Is the table warm enough? Or cool enough? One size does not fit all. Check with the client when you first re-enter the room for the massage, and again during the massage. When a client is cold they become tense, and contracted muscles do not release well.

Lie down on your own table occasionally to see how it feels. Did your face cradle get catawampus without you realizing it? If so your clients will feel it and you will want to know what they experience by checking it out for yourself from time to time. Better yet, get a massage in your own room on your own table. You will really get a good feel for what the client sees and feels in there.

By the way, we have all heard you can tell a lot about the quality of an office by the **plants** in the office. I respectfully disagree. I have a challenge of little natural light in my office which is not uncommon for massage therapy treatment rooms. I have tried several different plants with low requirements for light, but none of them thrived and most did not survive. As I did my best to keep them going, sometimes they looked pretty sickly. I was determined to keep trying, so I kept them in place longer than I probably should have. I am a fan of living plants and wanted their benefit of cleaning the indoor air. Eventually I gave up and I brought in a few very realistic silk plants that do bring their own appearance of life to the office.

If you **smoke,** refrain while at work unless all your clients are smokers. Or better yet, quit! Your clothing holds the odor of smoke and your clients can smell it even when you can't. Massage is health care and non-smoking clients do not like to breathe smoke while they are on the table. Enough said.

Are you **dressed appropriately**, in clean and modest attire? The clothing you choose says a lot about your practice, your personality, and your efforts. Professional looking clothing doesn't mean expensive and flashy, it means clean and appropriate. That's all. Some therapists wear scrubs and they look comfortable and professional at the same time. Scrubs come in all price ranges too. Others wear slacks that look nice and comfortable. For female therapists, never wear a revealing shirt, as this could send the wrong message. Remember, your image is as important as your technique!

Between clients **be ready** every time you answer the phone. Keep paper and pen out in the open on your desk or table so you can write down the caller's name and everything they tell you immediately as they are speaking. You will be able to call them by name right away. When you are able to ask detailed questions about the symptoms they have already described, they will know immediately you were listening. They will see you are a professional and ready to serve. They will realize you are paying attention to them already and will appreciate not having to repeat everything they just said. Some callers are shopping around for a therapist and may have some vague questions to see how you present yourself. When they start by asking about your prices, do you simply answer their questions or do you expand your opportunity to sell yourself? Take a little time to write out a few points about yourself, your practice, and the reasons why this caller should book an appointment with you. Can you quickly list a few benefits of massage in general? Do you have experience in their area of concern such as frozen shoulder or sore neck muscles? Telling a caller that you treat people with sore neck muscles every day, or you have recently seen three clients whose shoulder issues have improved, will help the prospective client feel confident in giving you a try.

Properly addressing the above areas conveys an attitude of service to the customer and shows your interest in their comfort. It also indicates your professionalism and your dedication to being the best and doing your best. Look for any other ways you can think of to treat your customers with excellence, and you will be rewarded with a successful practice and returning clients.

Keep Your Calendar With You Always

If you are serious about building a busy practice, you must keep your calendar with you everywhere you go with only two exceptions: bed and bath! Otherwise, always have it. You never know when you will receive a call, especially when you are not in your office, and you want to be ready to speak professionally with the caller and book them on the spot! I carried mine everywhere including the grocery store. If I received a call, I stopped my cart to give my caller my full attention. Sometimes they didn't even realize I was not in the office. If it was clear that I was in Aisle 6, I would simply apologize for the background noise and tell the caller they caught me on my day off. They appreciate even more that you answered your phone and helped them book an appointment. While you are at it, keep gift certificates with you too! You know how it happens. So often we intend to make a call, place an order, or buy a gift, and it gets put off. Well, you will hear it from clients and prospective clients too. You will be amazed at how often you will run into an acquaintance who says "I've been meaning to call you, I need a gift for my daughter". You can make the sale right then and there and everybody is happy and cared for. Do not let a potential sale get away because you were unprepared. You both win and go on with your day feeling happy!

Fake It Till You Make It

Earlier I referred to the phrase **'Fake it till you make it'**. It worked for me when I was beginning my practice, and here is how it works: When people call for appointments and ask "when do you have time available?" you do not have to say you haven't had one client yet this week. Seriously, in the early days, weeks, and months, you are likely to have more open time than filled appointments. I wasn't about to say "well,

I have 20 hours open this week, take your pick!" Without saying anything that wasn't true, my answer became "I have openings on Wednesday at 2:00, Friday at 10:30, and Saturday at 11:30. Will one of those work for you?" Mind you, there were other options. I took a gamble by picking out those openings in particular. I chose appointments I especially wanted to fill first, perhaps because they were before or after another appointment already booked. I chose what would work best with my schedule while giving the caller options, but I know that I also might have totally missed the mark. To help you make specific appointment suggestions for someone you don't know well, ask first if they need evening and weekend opportunities, or are they available during the work day. Almost always the person will offer details about their schedule, allowing us to target their availability and at the same time offer a time that would work best for us. Occasionally a caller would say their only day open is their day off, and that happened to be my day off too. I learned to think quickly if I could switch my off day. Listen to the difference in the dialog between the two methods:

Prospective Client: "I've been meaning to call you, Mary Alice. When do you have an opening for a one hour massage?"
Me: "Well, let me see (as I'm opening my calendar), are you available during the workday hours or do you need evenings and weekends?"
PC: "Oh my week is pretty full next week but I can come in most mornings after I take Lisa to Kindergarten, which is at 9 am."
Me: "Great! How about Tuesday?" (I know that I already have an 11:00 booked and if I can book this person at 9:30 that day I'll have two in a row, making my day more efficient.

      Doesn't that sound a lot more professional than "I have 20 hours open this week, take your pick"? Not only does it sound more professional, it doesn't give away the fact that you may be desperate for work. When clients know or at least think you are practicing regularly they will feel a greater level of confidence in your work.

Also, when either friends or clients asked me early on how business was, my answer was always **"It's going well!"** Other truthful answers could be "I am really glad I made this career choice," or "It takes a lot of my time, but I am really excited and passionate about what I do". Another good short answer is "business is growing". Four clients per week for the first six months is a good number so you are doing well! If they ask if my schedule is full, I truthfully answer that I still have room for more clients. It's nobody's business what the nitty gritty details are, and success begets more success. Speak prosperity and focus on prosperity! While five massages per week is not your ultimate definition of success, it is success in early times so it's all true. The number that defines success for you will change as time goes on and your experience grows, and the number of clients you see each week will grow. I believe in following the advice of Louise Hay who said, "Be grateful for what you do have and you will find that it increases."

Keep Detailed Notes

Whether you keep records on paper or electronically, keep them well. In addition to notes about the client's physical condition and all the medical information you need to keep current, include details such as the names of children, pets, plus any special interests and special dates. When a client's parent passes away, I make a note of that in the file and usually send them a card on the anniversary. People appreciate that kind of attention and compassion. You don't want any client to feel he or she is one of many, just part of a rotating number of people through the office every day. Have you ever visited a physician's office and ended up feeling this way? Who hasn't? With a full hour on the table plus a few minutes before and after the massage treatment, you have lots of opportunity to get to know your client in meaningful ways by listening to what they say and making notes to help you follow up.

Be sure to **review your previous notes** before the client's visit so you can properly anticipate their preferences such as extra warmth and if they like to chat during massage or have quiet. You will want to read what you worked on during his last visit and ask how he has progressed since then. If you have made a note of the techniques you tried or recommended he use at home, you will want to learn if they have been effective so you can continue on this course of action or suggest a new technique. And if she came in last visit excitedly telling you about her new puppy, you can call the puppy by name and ask how it is doing. Personal attention like this goes a long way in making a client feel special, cared for, and important to you, which of course they are!

Step by Step: Making a Massage Excellent

Your client's first visit is a critical time for you to make an excellent initial impression. Listening carefully, making and holding eye contact, asking pertinent questions, addressing their concerns, anticipating sensitive issues they may be reluctant to bring up, and in general being open, focused, and unhurried will all show the new client how much you care.

I start each first session by walking calmly toward the new client, establishing and holding eye contact while smiling and extending my hand in a gentle but firm handshake. I greet the person, let's call her Pam, and say "Hi Pam, I'm Mary Alice. Welcome." Right away Pam knows 1) she has my attention, 2) she is in the right place, and 3) I'm happy to see her. Then I build on this foundation by inviting Pam to sit in the rocking chair in my treatment room – a huge invitation to relax in itself while I lock the door between the waiting room and the hallway. Now Pam knows we can speak confidentially and we will not be disturbed. Here is my favorite surprise for new clients: I have warmed a shoulder/neck pillow and I ask Pam if I can place it on her shoulders while we talk. This offer is always met with a smile and usually a deep sigh. I can almost hear Pam's blood pressure going down!

I sit near Pam so we can speak in comfortable tones as this is all personal information. Rather than hand Pam a clipboard and ask her to record her information for me, I prefer to make this a conversation. I maintain eye contact, keep a calm manner and voice, and gently proceed through the medical history questions. Her answers tell me who she is, her past injuries, the physical and mental stressors she is dealing with now, and her goals for today's session and possible future sessions. All of these simple tactics reinforce my message that I care about Pam, and I want to help her feel better. I want her to know I am a professional who can make a difference. All this exchange of comfort, trust, and integrity and she is not even on the table yet!

One of my first questions is whether Pam has had a professional massage before and if so, approximately how long it has been since her last massage. This gives me an idea of the general condition of her muscles and how many toxins they may be holding, especially if it has been years since she had her last massage.

So now, let's assume this is Pam's first massage. She may not know what to expect or how to ask what happens next. Knowing it is Pam's first massage prompts me to offer details about the massage process that will certainly help her feel more relaxed. I explain briefly what comes next as we progress. Don't we all have some fear of the unknown? You can help your clients relax by anticipating their questions. I tell Pam that she may undress to her own level of comfort. She will be covered at all times while I expose only the part or limb on which I am working, one at a time. I instruct Pam whether I want her to be face up or face down on the table, and that I will leave the room for her to get on the table in private. I tell her I will knock on the door before entering the room again to be certain she is ready. Now here comes my second favorite tactic: before I leave the room for her to get undressed, I ask Pam if she has any questions for me. It is so simple, but so effective! How many times have you been with a health care provider who did all the talking and then left the room, leaving you frustrated and confused and feeling utterly unheard? Given the opportunity to ask whatever she is still unclear about, how could a client feel anything but comfortable when you are again showing her you are patient, compassionate, and truly care about her well-being?

Once she is situated on the table, I begin by telling Pam that this is her hour and she has the power to decide if she wants quiet or would prefer to talk during the massage. I tell her that I will have a few questions for her about my pressure or her comfort, but other conversation is entirely up to her. I know that some people truly relax more completely if they chat through the hour, and others prefer to get lost in the quiet and solitude of their treatment time. Keep in mind, however, that some clients might want to be quiet in one appointment, but then will want to chat more next time.

Since Pam is new to massage I'll briefly and **quietly explain what I'm doing** as I progress through the massage unless I sense – or she tells me – that she is quite comfortable, relaxed, and has given herself over to trusting in my care. I interrupt her peacefulness less as I detect more relaxation on her part.

What I don't say to clients is that I **open the session with a silent prayer** as I begin the massage and it goes something like this: "Thank You Heavenly Father for Your blessings on Pam. Thank You for blessing Pam with Your peace, Your love, and Your healing energy. Thank you for blessing Pam in whatever way she needs, according to Your will and Pam's highest good." I use this prayer for every client every day because I believe this prayer helps me focus on positive and healing energy in whatever way is appropriate for each client on this particular day.

When I ask a client for **feedback on the pressure** I'm using, I started out asking 'how is my pressure today"? That question can be harder to answer when the client either doesn't know what to expect or doesn't want to complain. Now I ask Pam "Would this feel better if I used more or less pressure?" This way she can easily say 'more' or 'less' and get what she wants and needs.

While **working on a client's neck** I am especially careful to be gentle and make slow movements so the client doesn't have to worry that I will hurt him or her. The neck is a critically important area. It is a common area of tension. Stay extra focused here to show respect to help the client relax so you can get into the muscles and encourage healing.
At the same time, I do my best to avoid spreading massage **oil or cream into the client's hair**. The client may be going back to work if this appointment is during daytime hours, or they may need to make stops on the way home from this appointment. Either way, most people prefer not to leave a massage feeling like their appearance is altered in a negative way. When I was new I worked on a lovely lady during an evening appointment. I knew she had come from work and was going home after the massage. I was not overly careful with oil on her neck or with her hair when I massaged her scalp. Well, after the massage when she came out of the room, I knew I was in trouble when the first thing she said was "look at my hair!" She clearly was not happy. I didn't see what the big deal was at the time, but I learned! She was genuinely unhappy that I had messed up her hair. She never came back. Do your best to use only the smallest amount of lubricant possible on the neck, keep as much as possible out of their hair, and your clients will be grateful. While you are at it, do your best to **be sure you are not pulling your client's hair**. Short hair and long hair can all be pulled to the point of

pain while working on the posterior neck if you are not careful, and that is an uncomfortable situation for any client.

I'm in the habit of asking the client when she turns over about the **temperature**. For a long time the question was exactly that: "How is the temperature for you?" Most of the time the answer I received was 'it's fine'. Now I've evolved that question to sound like this: "Pam, would you like the temperature adjusted up or down?" With this question she can easily respond with one word "up, down, or no" without sounding like she's complaining. Every time you make life easier for the client, they will appreciate you. Another thought about table warmers is how convenient they are for keeping the client warm without overheating the therapist. Using a warmer that is specifically made for massage tables, or getting a twin size heated mattress pad, is up to you, but I highly recommend using something. Otherwise you must keep the room far too warm for your own comfort, or the client will be cold and uncomfortable.

All during the massage, whether I find muscles that feel tight or when everything feels healthy, I often will silently say '**Peace be with you**'. I'm inviting blessings on this client in the way of peace, in and around her. Most of the time clients do not know I do this, but I do it for everyone. I also pray for each client during the massage, and again most clients do not know it. Occasionally a client will ask me to pray for them and give a specific reason, and then I always tell them that I pray every time I see them. Often this brings tears to their eyes. Who doesn't need and want to be prayed for?

If you truly desire to give your client an experience he or she will want to come back for, **don't plan to use your phone during the massage.** This may seem like a no-brainer, but it's not. It needs to be stated and heard, loud and clear. I have called other therapists to book an appointment, and when I stated the reason for my call, I have been asked "Can I call you back on that? I'm giving a massage right now". While

85

I could feel flattered that my call was answered, I don't because I think it is highly disrespectful to the client on the table who is paying for your time. I felt badly to have interrupted a massage. I assumed that the therapist would not answer if unavailable, and giving a massage means you are unavailable! Yes, we all know we never want to miss a call, but the nature of our business is to give our full attention to the person on the table right now. Your clients will appreciate the opportunity to leave a message on your voice mail when they know you will also let other calls go to voice mail when they are on the table. What would Pam think if I was giving her a great massage and stopped to answer the phone? How would you feel? I have also heard from a client who told me she was getting a one-handed massage while the therapist was texting with the other hand. The client could hear the clicking. Don't do it if you are serious about being a good massage therapist.

Of course, there are special circumstances, and on those days it is important to let your client know what is going on. When my son and daughter-in-law went to the hospital in labor 650 miles away, I wanted to keep my phone near me to hear the news as soon as possible. That day, I told each client the situation and asked if they minded if I had the phone in the room with us. All my clients were completely agreeable to this. I placed the phone on a table where I could see it without touching it, and the ringer was turned off so it would only vibrate softly if the call I was waiting for came in during the massage. When the phone buzzed for other callers, I was able to see who it was and wait until later to deal with them without disturbing my current client. It became almost a game as each client wanted to be the one on the table when the all important call finally came!

Are you a **clock watcher**? I never was before becoming a massage therapist, but I changed that quickly. Keeping an eye on the time throughout the massage will help you give a balanced treatment. Knowing where you want to spend extra time before you start, and keeping track of where you are and what you still want to accomplish, will keep you from spending too much time in any one area and having to rush through all the parts you didn't get to yet. Plan out your course of action for each massage, and follow it closely while being on the lookout for any trouble spots you may find that require a little more attention. You can enjoy the peacefulness of the massage you are giving right along with your client who ends up feeling balanced and whole.

Here's another trick I use daily: when I look at the clock early in the hour I'll say the time to myself and add 'and **all is well**'. Then as the time is winding down and I'm trying to be sure I have time to include everything I had planned for this client, I look at the clock, see that I have eight minutes left, and say to myself: 'Eight minutes left and all is well. What still needs to be done?' I don't want to pass up any opportunity to invite wellness into this room and onto this client. This is one more way I can feel like I'm doing everything I can to encourage health.

As I move about the treatment room during a massage, I do my best to **be as quiet and gentle as possible**. Have you ever been on a massage table, fully relaxed and floating somewhere above the clouds, completely forgetting where you are at this moment, only to have the therapist bump into the table and jar you abruptly back to reality? Whether a client comes in for treatment of a frozen shoulder or to let go of the week's tension, there comes a time in the massage when they are able to check out mentally. We can help them get to that point more quickly and stay there longer, enhancing the relaxation effect, by being quiet and gentle. Don't make unnecessary noise with bottles of oil or the towel warmer as you open and close the door. Don't sniff or cough all through the massage. The quieter you are, the better you are able to hear your client's breathing and the sooner you will know it if Pam is holding her breath because something hurts! Regardless of the reason they have come in for massage, we want our clients to be able to relax fully and float away if they want to. They may look like they are just resting on your table but mentally, emotionally, and nearly physically they may be gone to their favorite beach or lake house, watching the sunset with a virtual glass of wine or tea. One therapist I see occasionally takes this to the next level of complete respect for his clients. When he needs to ask me something during my massage, he always prefaces his question by quietly and gently saying "Mary Alice, I'm sorry to interrupt you (I'm not talking, mind you), is this spot tender?" I love that! I feel so respected! His kindness inspires me to be as kind as possible to my clients. Remember that people may forget what you said or did, but they will never forget how you made them feel.

When the appointment **time is almost over** and you feel you need to spend an extra five or ten minutes to complete your treatment plan, don't go over without speaking up. Ask the client if you will make them late for any appointments if you go over by five or ten minutes. Usually the client will say no, but sometimes they will be short on time and need to get moving soon. That's when the client will really appreciate your consideration for their time. The client is also likely to appreciate your giving them a little extra time without charge. Showing that your attention is on their health and well-being rather than a strict adherence to time will win points for you every time!

Once I visited an experienced therapist for the first time. We chatted easily and she was very good at finding tension in my muscles and releasing it. Her office was calm, her music peaceful, and her style comforting. I felt comfortable and well attended throughout the massage treatment. When she left the room and I got up to get dressed, however, I learned that she had gone thirty minutes over our expected one-hour massage. This was generous of her but I had a plane to catch! Immediately I was in stress mode and all her excellent work was erased. Don't waste your time and your client's time and money! The person on the table has no concept of the amount of time that is passing, so be kind and ask if you need to go over the agreed amount of time.

At the end of a massage I use another **silent prayer** that sounds like this: "May the White Light of God surround Pam and keep out all negative energy. May Pam live in peace, joy, health, prosperity, alignment, balance, compassion, contentment, and surrounded by true love. And so it is. Thanks be to God. Lord Jesus you are the source of love, compassion, and healing, and I am Your willing instrument. Amen." I believe that we are the hands of God and He is the healer. The more we thank Him for bringing healing energy to ourselves and our clients, I believe the more we are open to receive His healing energy.

At the conclusion of the treatment session, I gently place my hand on the client's upper back if she is prone, on her shoulder if she is supine, and quietly tell her to take her time and be careful getting off the table. If she is a first timer like Pam, I tell her I'll be leaving the room so she knows she will be free to dress again in private. Then I instruct the client to either come out into the outer office when ready, or to open the door and I'll come back in when he or she is ready. We conclude the session in private so any questions can be addressed, payment takes place, and the next appointment is discussed.

Stay focused on your client during this ending time. Watch your tone of voice and keep it calm and soothing. Make eye contact, listen to the client, and show him or her you are listening by responding thoughtfully. Ask questions if appropriate. Even if you know you want to get going, either to prepare for the next client or to go home, never act in a way as to give the client the impression you are in a hurry. You want him or her to keep that peaceful feeling as long as possible don't you? Smile and be peaceful.

Once Pam has left the office, next comes cleaning the room and re-setting the table for the next client. You know what that means? **Laundry!** We do a lot of laundry, and it goes with the territory. Accept it as a fact of life. If you are in an office situation where you have laundry facilities on site, fantastic! Even better if laundry tasks are someone else's job to perform, provided the linens come back to you as clean and soft as you like them to be. When you have total control over your laundry, you get to choose whether to use unscented or scented products, and which brands you prefer. This is important if you have clients with sensitive skin. If you must take your laundry home, I understand completely how you feel. It can be daunting at times when you are tired or ready to move on to another activity. Therefore, there is only one way to look at a pile of laundry – as prosperity! Be thankful for your prosperity as you are taking care of your linens.

Finally, follow up the first appointment with a hand-written, personal **thank-you note** sent through the old-fashioned mail. Many clients have told me that note was really appreciated. It's a nice touch, in my opinion, again demonstrating your commitment to personally caring for your clients, and it can be the final detail that sets you apart from the others. My thank-you note includes a sentence thanking the client for coming to me for massage therapy, an expression of the benefits of massage that matches this person's own concerns, and a request that she call me if she has any questions, or when she is ready for her next massage treatment.

You have now set the bar pretty high for what all clients can expect from massage therapy. Picture this: if Pam goes to another therapist next time, for whatever reason, and she is not treated with all this kindness, whom do you think she will call after that? Clients will drive longer distances to get to you when they like your style and the way you treat them.

Keep in Mind...

Do not make **promises** about results. We cannot guarantee anything in particular. We can estimate how the client might feel over the next 24 to 48 hours by saying 'In the past, clients have told me they felt a little sore for the first day, but it went away after that and they felt much better'. More than anything you say, the massage you just gave will build the client's confidence in you. If you have done your best to treat her with complete respect, paid close attention to your pressure, and given her a balanced massage, she will know she can relax and trust you.

When I was still in massage school I had a potential client ask me how school was going and why I enjoyed it. She had never experienced massage. She confided that she has an issue with constipation. We had recently studied abdominal massage and its effectiveness was impressed upon the class, so much that several of us came to class the night of the practice session wearing very easy off clothing in fear that we would have to make a mad dash to the rest room! Remember that class? We learned that it works well but not quite that fast (thankfully!), and I arrogantly answered yes when this prospective client asked if I could guarantee results for her. Really, we can't guarantee anything, but I was sure it would work! Well, she did not book an appointment and never again brought up the possibility of massage. I often wondered if I had answered her differently if she might have given it a try. Perhaps I could have said our massage teachers impressed upon us that this technique is very effective. The only way to see what kind of results she would experience would be to give it a try. Since I was still in school, I would then have the opportunity to remind her that the session would be free of charge, so there was nothing to lose. If only...but remember we are all going to make mistakes. Forgive yourself and remember the lesson.

If applicable, give the client **self-care instructions** for home use between massage sessions. Is there a stretch you know will help? Maybe a breathing exercise? Do you think heat therapy will continue or expand the healing that you have begun? Helping your clients feel good, heal, and be their best always and not just when they are on the massage table, shows them that you truly care about their health and well-being. At first glance, it might seem that you gain nothing for helping them take care of themselves at home, but think again. You are conducting yourself as a true healing professional, not just a massage therapist for hire. Also, we know that monthly massage is not going to be enough to balance out the 10 hours this client is working on a computer daily if he doesn't do some stretching during the month. And if he does the stretching you advise, then the next massage he gets will help him that much more because he is coming from a place of more comfort rather than extreme pain. Win-win.

Two questions I have heard often from new clients are "**How long will it take to fix this?**" and "**How often do you recommend getting massage?**" I think these two questions go together because while you can't necessarily predict how quickly they will heal, you can talk about the benefits of, and your past success with, several therapy sessions closely timed. You can follow up with encouragement in preserving their well-being in the future and preventing a return of pain. Regular massage when a client feels good is an excellent tool for preventing tight muscles from creeping up and surprising us with "sudden" pain that "comes out of nowhere". The client's goal today may be to solve the pain they feel or the tension that is restricting their movement. Our opportunity here is to speak to their long term goals of staying healthy, being strong, maintaining flexibility, and being comfortable. Encouraging a client to come in weekly for four weeks, and then re-evaluating if sessions can be spread out, is not about promoting ourselves as therapists. In reality we are showing that we are focused on them and their health and well-being. If we can think in terms of how our services help them, not how desperate we are to fill our schedule, it becomes so much easier to talk about what we offer and invite them to come back regularly.

When I was just starting out, one of my most difficult moments was after the massage and payment when I wanted to ask the client if he would like to **book his next appointment**. How can I ask that? Isn't that presumptuous of me? Pushy? You might be feeling the same way. Many of my classmates expressed this same concern. Our teachers did a good job of telling us we are actually being helpful to our clients by asking them to book again, but it certainly didn't feel that way in the beginning. It was just too scary since I was also aware of the financial implications for me. Now I can tell you that our teachers were absolutely right. It's not so hard once you get more comfortable with the whole business. Give it some thought and develop a sentence or two that feels right to you. Role play and actually practice it with an imaginary client sitting in front of you. Once I came up with mine, I was able to ask virtually everyone and quickly became comfortable with the task. My question went like this: "Do you prefer to call when you are ready to book your next massage, or book it now so you know you have it on your calendar to look forward to it?" I still use this question for new clients. Many will book again right then, and it helps me get to know them even better. Of course I make a note of this preference in their file.

It's All Confidential

During the taking of the medical history I always tell the client that everything we talk about is completely **confidential**. If the client and I have a mutual friend or acquaintance, I usually will assure them that even if the friend asks about our visit, I will not give out any details other than to say that our visit went well. I think it is important to say this clearly and directly to the client, even though it is posted on my web site and on the consent form, so that the client knows I am serious about confidentiality. As therapists it is our duty to maintain confidentiality at all costs. Massage is a very personal business and it is not easy for some clients to let their physical imperfections be seen or for them to share their thoughts. Clients will often open up and start talking during the massage about something that has been on his or her mind. Several times I have had this happen and a few minutes later, when the client realized she said more than she intended, she added "I don't usually talk so openly about this". That is our cue as therapists to assure the client that confidentiality is the rule and whatever they say will go no further. There is no substitute for professionalism here, and a breach of confidentiality often cannot be repaired. Respect your clients at all times by remembering how important it is to the client to know he or she can depend on you.

Do You Have the Heart of a Teacher?

One of the most important keys I have found for building a successful massage therapy practice is taking on the role of **teacher**. Our clients look to us for information and it is very important for us as professionals to teach our clients about health and well-being. If a new client calls to book an appointment and asks you if you can help his shoulder pain, what is the first thing you can do to show him you are a professional? Ask a few questions. This is the simplest but most important step in creating rapport with this new person and beginning the education process. What actually is going on with his shoulder: was there an accident? Is this a sports injury? Has he been painting a house? Does he work on a computer 80 hours per week? How long has he felt the pain? Asking questions like these will give you a lot more information and lead you to serving each client well. You will also show him that you know enough to narrow down the answer to his question to be specific to his needs. Your goal is to solve his problem, and you can only find out the source of his problem if you ask questions. If the caller is in pain and it will be several hours or even a day or two before you can see him, is there something you can suggest he do while he is waiting that might bring him some relief? Once the client comes in and you get a better idea of what he is dealing with, turn that information into stretches or warming techniques that the client can do at home between massages. Teaching a client about self-care between massages shows you are interested in them, in their health and well-being, and not just how many clients you can squeeze in per day to increase your income.

Here is a question that will come up more often indirectly but sometimes directly too, and if you give it some thought now you will be ready with an answer regardless of how it is presented to you. Is the massage you give for **relaxation** or is it **therapeutic massage**? This is an excellent opportunity to teach our clients that all massage is good for them. I talk about the fact that I give relaxing massages, but that doesn't make them "fluff" massages or any less therapeutic. We learn in massage school that the body heals and all systems work much better when we are relaxed and the parasympathetic nervous system is working efficiently rather than being in a state of stress with cortisol and any other stress hormones running rampant. Massage can solve a pain or tension issue and be relaxing at the same time. With all the prayer, focus on health and well-being, and peace that I invite during massage, I believe what I do is true health care. I am caring for the health of every person I treat. I encourage more health with massage techniques. I invite healing. I invite peace and balance. Massage may seem, to many people at first, to be on the level of pampering, but it is also serious business in promoting the health of the client. In my opinion, all massage is therapeutic, regardless of the reason that brought the client in for treatment. And I believe that all massage can be relaxing, again regardless of what brought the client in for treatment. In reality, the answer is both. Massage is an excellent opportunity to slow down, find balance, and be well.

Client Gifts

I think it is helpful to let your clients know you **appreciate** them with occasional tokens of that appreciation. I have been known to give a small gift to my most regular clients sometime between Thanksgiving and Christmas. It's not meant to be a Christmas gift as such, but an appreciation gift. In the past I have included cards mentioning my thankfulness for their business and my wish for blessings on them and their family. For the first few years I did some kind of promotion during National Massage Therapy Week. One year I gave a relaxing music CD to each person who got a massage that particular week. I was able to buy the CD's at a quantity discount so it didn't cost an extraordinary amount for me, and my clients enjoyed the bonus. If you are short on funds but long on time, you might offer an extra 15 minutes free for each 60 minute massage booked that week. I've also given Client Appreciation cards that included a coupon for $10 off a 60 minute massage in January. What a great way to encourage a client to come in for their regular massage after the hustle and bustle of the holidays and save a little money too. For many years I sent birthday cards to clients offering them their choice of a discount on their hour massage or extra time for free. Clients looked forward to receiving that card and appreciated the extra time or the savings. I do appreciate business my clients give me and I want them to know it.

Your talent is God's gift to you. What you do with it is your gift back to God.

Leo Buscaglia

Part Three

The Private Practice

If you want to start your own small business, you can't expect anyone else to do the work for you. The key ingredient in small business is you. You are the energy, dreams, and passions.

Dave Ramsey

Following the suggestions contained in *Table Manners* will help you set yourself apart from other therapists regardless of where you work. By practicing excellence in all you do, clients will soon be asking for you by name when they call to book an appointment at the spa, resort, salon, or office where you work. Success can be yours regardless of your place of practice.

Working for someone else has many benefits. The establishment will handle most of the marketing of the business, and they may do all your scheduling and laundry. In addition, you will not be required to pay rent, utilities, and furnish your space. However, there is a price to be paid for all of this being done for you, and you are free to decide what you prefer according to your skills and comfort level. Being in private practice poses additional challenges as well as rewards, and it truly is not for everyone. In private practice you are actually the owner and operator of a business.

Being on your own is an exhilarating, frightening, liberating, lucrative, exhausting, satisfying adventure! There is nothing like it! While you get to maintain control of your practice to a much greater degree than working for someone else, not to mention keeping a larger portion of the income, there are more aspects on the business side that require great knowledge, initiative, and diligence. This is where you really get to shine though! Sometimes it will seem like the task list will never end. It will. Take it one day at a time. Do your best to take good care of all the details. Work really hard for as long as it takes in the beginning to get everything up and running, and over time you will be able to relax and enjoy what you have created. Use the following as a checklist for serious consideration and attention.

1. **Take plenty of time when setting up your website** and consider carefully how the information is displayed and could be viewed by all prospective clients. Put your contact information on every page so the reader can easily click on the page of information most important to her and so she already has your phone number right in front of her. I have often been

frustrated by viewing a web site, gathering necessary information, then had to look through several more pages to find how to contact the person or company. Let's make it easy for them to pick up the phone and call us.

2. **Add to your web site pictures or graphics you really like that reflect the peace and serenity of your practice.** Make sure you use a picture or two that are actually taken in your treatment room. If you use peaceful and lovely landscapes for some of the decorations on your web site, that will certainly add to the calming effect for readers, but don't use spa pictures that are not your own, leading to disappointment when the client thinks she knows what your treatment room looks like and finds out it is totally different.

3. **Include client testimonials and lots of details on your site.** Prospective clients look for reviews by other clients and customers. Include any special services you offer like warm pillows, a table warmer, paraffin hand dip, and the like. Clearly spell out your prices for each service, specifying what is free or included in the price of an hour massage. Do you go out to businesses for chair massage? Add a page for that information. You never know when a prospective client may be inspired to book you for a visit to the office. If you offer a newsletter to your clients, be sure to include instructions for how to subscribe to it. In some places an hour massage is actually 50 minutes on the table. If your hour massage is a full 60 minutes on the table, let everyone know it!

4. **Develop a brochure.** Include all your policies, your mission statement, guiding principles, credentials, rates, schedule, menu of services, and everything else you want people to know about you. It will be almost a paper version of your website, but not completely. Refer people to your website for more information. You will need these brochures to hand out at charity events, meetings, and marketing opportunities of all types. Keep it simple and clear. One double-sided page is probably best. The cost will be

reasonable and you can fold it for easy transport. With an affordable color printer at home or in your office you can plan to print your own brochures for at least the first few years. You'll constantly be adding to it as your practice develops and you learn new modalities. Print 10 or 20 at a time in the beginning to keep waste to a minimum. You can make it look professional while keeping it simple and excellently informative for all prospective clients.

5. **When a current client refers a friend** who comes to see you, do you offer a referral reward of $10 off their next massage or ten minutes free to the referring client? Spell that out on your web site too. Since referrals are our best advertisements, clients will appreciate receiving a bonus when they send a friend to you for treatment. Readers will see how thorough you are in presenting the important details of your practice and they will know that you have done it thoughtfully. By anticipating most or all of their possible questions, you are making it easy for anyone to contact you.

6. **Represent your skills properly** in your brochures, on your web site, in your office where you display your credentials, and in every conversation about how you can help your clients. If you have studied a technique, let your clients know. If you feel confident that you can help a client with the issue they describe, say so. Speak up if you have seen the issue before and the client's pain was reduced or resolved. Be careful not to state or even imply actual certification in any technique unless you truly are certified. Many times certification is not required to be able to use a technique you have learned.

7. **Consider offering a wellness plan.** That's what I call a series of massages that are offered at a discount provided the treatment is received within a relatively short period of time. When I met a lovely lady who was about to see a surgeon for a shoulder issue, and she experienced significant relief with just one massage session, she was very

interested in coming back soon to see what else massage could do for her. At that time I gave her the option to receive four 60-minute massages for the price of three if she booked them now, either two or four weeks apart. In order to see what healing we could achieve we needed to have the treatments close together to compound the benefits. She was delighted with the discount and with the results of massage. Her shoulder surgery was cancelled and never needed. One prospective client bought a wellness package for his wife when he probably would have bought only a one hour gift certificate. A wellness plan is a great way to encourage new clients to come back, learn how massage can help them, and learn about you as a therapist at least in the early years. After I was in practice about six years and my schedule stayed pretty full, I discontinued offering the wellness package. It was no longer necessary to discount my work and I was showing respect for myself by charging full price now. I never did formally advertise this wellness plan because I didn't want to offer it across the board. I offered it verbally when I sensed that a new client would benefit from it. I had several people use it consistently for several years in the beginning and we both benefited from it: they got into the routine of regular massage and found out how good they could feel, and I had more people on my schedule.

8. **Stay with your favorite schedule.** I leave 30 minutes open between appointments and advertise my practice as a No Stress Zone. If clients are running a little early or a little late, they know they will still get their full time without anyone rushing dangerously to get to my office. Scheduling that way leaves plenty of time for a client's questions too. I benefit from this timing also since I can take care of myself better with time between clients to breathe, get a drink, or return a phone call.

9. **Consider writing a monthly newsletter** for your clients. I started mine right away, while I had time to give it lots of thought, and called it "Be Well". Be Well is more than a

name—it is my constant wish for my clients. It is also a thought I want to keep in front of my clients throughout the month. Clients have told me they post the newsletter on the refrigerator for reference or inspiration. Besides being a service to my client base, I feel the newsletter is an excellent opportunity to keep my name in front of clients, especially if it has been a while since they came to see me. Yes it takes some planning, time, and work, but I really think this is another tool that pays off big dividends. Keep in touch with everyone who has come to see you through a newsletter, either electronically, on paper, or some of each. I use both methods because some people prefer to have a paper copy to take out on the porch and read with a glass of tea. Give it some serious thought.

10. **Set your prices carefully and thoughtfully**. Present your services as high quality. Set your fees according to what you feel is fair. Offer discounts and specials in the early years to bring in more business. Do you want to offer discounts or a sliding payment scale for a particular population such as military veterans? Is this the population you want to focus on? Again, decide ahead so you will be ready. Consider carefully whether you want to advertise this formally or only verbally. Advertise if you want to, but be careful not to appear desperate for clients. You also don't want to attract too many clients who call only when you have a special promotion. One by one over time, phase out most discounts as your schedule fills up. If a client asks for a discount you have discontinued, gently but firmly say "I no longer discount my work because I've gained a lot of experience and my schedule stays rather full." Making a good and sustainable income by charging what you need to charge and not offering too many discounts actually helps clients, paradoxically. Low prices don't help clients, only fair prices. It's a win-win situation again. When a business charges too low prices and goes out of business, it hurts clients/customers because the business is no longer there to serve them.

11. **Decide how you'll handle late clients** because it will happen. Sometimes people are coming from work and traffic can slow them down. Perhaps the boss wanted to ask a few questions just before they left the office. Maybe a meeting goes long. Maybe a babysitter was late because her volleyball practice went long. Late happens and there are many legitimate reasons. I don't want anyone feeling frantic to get to my office on time and get into a traffic accident. Therefore, I schedule 30 minutes between massages. I advertise this through my newsletter so they know we have some flexible time. It gives us both a level of comfort and room to breathe. Also, clients sometimes have questions before or after their treatment. Giving them a few extra minutes can make the difference between a good massage and a great appointment. Most people appreciate our compassion especially if they are stressed by being late. I recommend treating them with respect and kindness, and rarely will anyone take advantage and be late on purpose!

12. **Record keeping** is critical for you as a small business. You must keep track of your income and deductable business expenses, resulting in extra paper work. Once you set up a system it is not too cumbersome, provided it is updated daily and summarized monthly. You will be sending in estimated tax payments quarterly to your state and federal government. Electronic options are available and simplify the tasks for you once you learn to use them. Take the time you have available in the early days to set up an efficient system and keep it current. You will be well prepared when tax time rolls around. Also, with monthly totals for expenses and income, you will be able to measure your progress and watch your success grow.

13. **Join a local business organization**. Networking with other professionals in your community is helpful in several ways. You will make new friends. You will learn of opportunities to market yourself to your community. You will learn of services that could be useful to your practice. Being

connected to other local professionals will boost your confidence.

14. **Plan for retirement**! While you are setting up a system to save money for estimated tax payments, also set up a savings account to build your nest egg. Self-employed workers do not have an employer-run savings program. It is up to you to make it happen. Get into the habit of contributing to your retirement savings regularly so you will be prepared when the time comes.

Private practice is rewarding and demanding at the same time. There is a lot to do and to think over carefully. If you really want to be your own boss, though, I say go for it! Make your decisions well and enjoy your freedom. Make your office space comfortable so you will look forward to spending your working hours there. Set your schedule the way it suits you best. Make everything your own and enjoy it every day!

I don't know what your destiny will be, but one thing I know; the only ones among you who will be really happy are those who will have sought and found how to serve.

Albert Schweitzer

Part Four

Handling Challenging Situations

If we could first know where we are…we could then better judge what to do, and how to do it.

Abraham Lincoln

Challenges in and to your practice will present themselves quickly when you are new, regardless of where you work. Address each problem or question immediately with curiosity, respect, and confidence as soon as you become aware of it. "Problems" indicate that you are making progress and learning. A variety of clients are being drawn to you. Awesome! If you don't have any problems or challenges, you might not be moving forward, which is the only way to go if you want to be a success. Standing still doesn't get you off square one. It might be comfortable, but it will get boring before long.

One example of a challenging situation is the client who repeatedly will call at the last minute to cancel, postpone, or just doesn't show up. Another example is when a client continues to talk for 20 minutes after the massage, payment, and next appointment booking are completed. We have already discussed the client who wants an appointment when you are not available in the boundaries section. There are also the occasional clients who don't understand that massage therapy is health care and not to be confused with the old term 'massage parlor'. I will give you a few suggestions here, but again I encourage you to also find other therapists in your geographical area to go to when any of these situations arise in your practice and you need immediate guidance.

Mentors

If you don't already have a **mentor** or a network of experienced therapists to whom you can go with questions, find someone now! Invest some time in getting to know people who can become your safety net. Your massage teachers, fellow classmates, practicing therapists in your area, and your local massage therapy association are all excellent sources for building your network. Colleagues with more experience than you will become priceless supports to you in the coming months.

I started going to massage therapy association meetings and found other therapists whom I could call as needed. They taught me so much! I also went to a different experienced therapist once or twice each year and took copious notes about absolutely everything from the way their rooms were set up and how they asked medical history questions to how they worked on my neck when I said it was a little stiff. Every therapist I met didn't become my mentor, but every one of them taught me more about what I wanted in my practice (and sometimes what I didn't want!)

Becoming a mentor to new therapists has been a priceless experience for me as well. New therapists constantly reminded me of muscles and techniques I had already forgotten about, and their questions helped me remember what I learned. The networking possibilities are endless when you make friends with other therapists, and your experience will be so much richer for the time you invest in getting to know therapists of all levels of experience.

Last Minute Changes/Cancellations

It can be unnerving when a **client doesn't show up** or calls at the last minute to say she has to work late and she wants to change her appointment. In the early months especially you want every single client to show up, be happy, and pay you! Realistically, clients are people first and they have many demands on their time and attention. I personally find it is important to be compassionate and as flexible as possible. No, we don't like it when we had the room all warmed up and ready and now we have no one to work on! Usually it helps to gently remind the client that you have reserved this hour exclusively for them. Let them tell you what happened to prevent their getting to the appointment. Show that you care about them by listening and commenting without being critical in your thoughts or your words. Most people are considerate and will not want this to happen again! If it does, my best advice is to study the situation case by case and determine if stronger action needs to be taken. I went so far as to send an invoice to a client who cancelled at the last minute repeatedly or just didn't show up. I didn't hear from her for a while and she did not pay the invoice. I think she got the message, however, because when she came back she always showed up at the appointed time or called well in advance to change her appointment. I think her time and attention were just stretched too far because she was working and going to school at the time. She is an excellent client again and we are both happy to see each other. Win-win.

The Cancellation Policy

Emergencies are always exceptions whether it's a sick client, the client has a sick child, there's a transportation issue, or the like. Clients appreciate it when we understand that getting a massage isn't the only thing on their calendar today.

What about situations where there is no emergency? It works out well to be lenient but firm. Your time is valuable so this is a really important point. Whatever you decide to set as your policy, post this information on your website and also in your treatment room. I have found it is helpful to call the client ten minutes after the appointed time if they have not arrived. Since I have no way of knowing yet if there is a true emergency, or if I have the appointment wrong, I like to leave the door open to either possibility. Regardless of whether I reach their voicemail or reach them directly, my first question is about their well-being: "I'm calling to see if you are okay because I had you on my schedule today for a 2:00 massage. Perhaps I wrote the appointment on the wrong date or at the wrong time." I would always prefer to err on the side of caution rather than accuse them of abusing my time. I don't want my clients to feel like they need to become defensive.

After all, mistakes happen. It might be my mistake or it might be their mistake. Either way, there is no use in pointing fingers or getting upset. What is important is finding out what happened so it can be corrected. If this client hasn't shown up today and her calendar says her appointment is tomorrow at 2:00, I need to know this! We need to get this straight so I am anticipating her visit and she knows I'm ready for her and no one else. Our goal is to have the person call back and come back. I'd prefer to foster an atmosphere of 'how can we solve this' rather than sound like 'you missed, you owe me'.

Now there are times when the client will say "Oh my word, I completely forgot! I knew this morning that our appointment was today and then I got busy and it slipped my mind." Here is where a large dose of diplomacy is important. If this is their first time, you might want to consider reviewing the cancellation policy with them. This policy should be posted in the office and on your web site. Explain that you understand these things happen and since it's the first time, you will be happy to overlook it. This clearly sends the message of THIS TIME you'll overlook it. For most people, they will be so happy you were forgiving that it will never happen again. If it does happen again, they usually will offer to pay for the missed session without you asking because they know that is fair and you have been lenient with them.

Alternately you can post your policy as "other than emergencies, if you miss your appointment please take responsibility to pay full price", and hope they take responsibility without you saying anything.

Long ago I had a client who missed two appointments in a row. When I called her after the first miss, I reached her voicemail and left the message I described above. Several hours later I learned she had sent me an email an hour before her appointment stating that she had to work later than expected. I prefer a phone call in this situation, but at least she tried. I asked her to call rather than email in the future. The second time she missed I called her and she said she had to work late again. I thought it was odd that I could hear party/bar noise clearly around her. I was kind about it, but I

113

couldn't afford to let this go on without speaking up for myself. In order to make my point, I asked her to consider how she would feel if she was sitting at her desk and her boss said he didn't have anything for her to do for the next hour. He would be back with more work in an hour so he needed her to stay in the office, but he wouldn't be paying her for this hour. This client understood my position after I spelled it out this way and we never had this problem again.

The Chatty Clients

Most likely every therapist will have a few **clients who want to visit** so much that their hour is just not enough time with you. Cool! But not so cool when you have another client due in 10 minutes and you need to get the room ready. Often this client is not being unkind or inconsiderate, they just like you! That's a good thing. Once I realize our conversation has spilled over into my time to prepare for the next client, I will usually stand up while looking at the person and listening to what they are saying. That often gives them the message that we must move on, and they will stand up and move toward leaving. If they don't seem to get it, I will interject when I get the chance that I am sorry but I have another client due soon. If the situation goes that far the client usually shows remorse and apologizes while hurrying to wrap up and be on their way. I never want the client to feel badly, so I maintain eye contact and a smile so they know I am not trying to be rude and I don't think they are rude. I am interested in them and what they have to say, but we have to move on.

More Than Massage

As for the people who are looking for **more than therapeutic massage**, being ready is your best defense so that it doesn't ruin your day, your attitude, or your practice. This is where experienced therapists will be more helpful than you can anticipate, as it seems we are all inevitably destined to be tested at least once. Having a trusted associate or mentor to talk with is extremely helpful. When it happened to me, I wasn't ready because it happened so early after I opened my practice. It really upset me. This client actually grabbed my hands and tried to place them where I wasn't going, ever! I was so shocked that he would do that but I simply said "I don't work there", and moved on. However, I was steaming and shaking on the inside. Afterward I questioned myself and what I had done wrong. Fortunately, I came to the conclusion that I did not do anything wrong!

This was one of those times in the early months that I was really glad I didn't have a lot of massages scheduled one after the other so I had time to calm down and talk with an experienced therapist to understand what had just happened. Once I could see the situation more calmly and clearly, I felt better able to deal with it. I called this client a few days later to tell him that I was cancelling his next appointment. I hoped I would reach his voicemail. Not only did he answer, but he asked why I was cancelling his appointment. Clearly in his mind he did nothing wrong. I calmly stated that I was not comfortable working with him. That was the end of my contact with this particular client.

No one has ever grabbed my hands again and the experienced therapists I checked with had never had this specific issue happen to them. Hearing this made me feel better because I didn't have to worry that this was a common occurrence. It took a little time, thought, talking with peers, and a fair amount of prayer, but I was able to relax and let go of any fear of running into this type of client again. Here are some of the changes I made to my practice to safeguard myself as much as possible:

A) Any time I receive a call from a male client who gives me even the slightest reason to doubt that he is looking for medical massage, I utilize this affirmation: "I love my appropriate clients". My intention is always to draw to me the appropriate clients without spending any time or energy on fearing inappropriate requests. Keep your statements – even to yourself – positive. Never let fear take over. Interestingly enough, about half of the times I felt unsure of a new client and used this affirmation, the client didn't show up for his appointment. I believe the universe took care of me. The other half of the time the client turned out to be completely fine. We do not want to be afraid to answer the phone and take on new clients. We just want to weed out the people who are looking for anything other than appropriate massage.

B) When a new male client booked an evening appointment a few months after this incident, I invited a trusted male relative to be present in the office during the client's appointment time. I didn't feel this was necessary for every new male client, but one gave me a slight inkling that all might not be well. The mere presence of someone in the office gave me a feeling of security. The client was completely fine and even became a regular client for years. I am so glad I didn't automatically turn him down because of fear!

C) My medical history form ends with the client signing that he or she is giving informed consent for treatment. Above the signature area is a list of my policies, and I verbalize them at the time we are completing the history form. I also suggest that the client take time to read the policies fully if he or she wishes. One policy clearly stated on this form, on my brochure, and on my website is "No sexual contact or implications are included in massage therapy here".

D) One other time I answered my phone on a Sunday evening while relaxing at home. Like many people these days, my mobile phone is the only phone I have. The number that appeared on my phone screen was from another state where I have extended family, so I thought this was going to be a personal call. That is the only reason I answered it. Normally I have learned not to answer my phone later in the evening or on the weekend unless I know who is calling. Keep in mind that legitimate callers often plan to leave a message when they know we probably are not in the office but they have time to call right now. They know they can accomplish this task regardless of the day or time. By letting us know of their interest, we can call them back when we are in the office again. They do not expect us to answer the phone at all hours of the day or night.

This time, however, not only was it not an extended family member calling, it was a man asking how many "ladies" I have for him and his friends. I was thankful he was so obvious in his request and I was confidently ready for him. I calmly and clearly stated that he had reached a medical massage practice and we are not open on Sunday evening. He thanked me and was gone. Easy enough.

E) For a while I kept my cell phone and my office keys in my pocket when I worked on a new male client in the evening. It gave me an extra level of security knowing that if I ever felt threatened I could leave the office quickly and have with me the most important items I would need to get help. I never had to use them, but I knew I was ready if a scary situation ever arose.

F) Many times I would turn on the lights and the music in another treatment room, and close the door. My client would have no idea if someone else was present or not. The appearance is there, however, that someone else is present. Often that is all it takes to prevent a situation from developing.

Any time you find yourself in an uncomfortable situation, maintain your composure and stay calm so you can think clearly. You will want to treat yourself and your caller or visitor with respect as long as possible. He doesn't necessarily want to hurt you; he just wants something you do not offer. Relax and let go of fear. The blessings of massage therapy are many and this can be an extremely fulfilling profession when you see clients improve with the appropriate therapy you provide. Don't ever let fear be your guiding factor. I love the way David Foster addresses this in *Accept No Mediocre Life*: "Fear adds up your short comings, subtracts from strengths, multiplies your worries, and divides your mind. It is powerful enough to blind you to opportunities as well as paralyze your hope and disengage your will." If I am tempted to give into fear, I repeat my mantra "I love my appropriate clients".

The credit belongs to the man who is actually in the arena; whose face is marred by dust, and sweat, and blood; who strives valiantly; who errs and comes short again and again; who knows the great enthusiasm, the great devotions, and spends himself in a worthy cause; who at the best knows in the end the triumph of high achievement; and who at worst, if he fails, at least he fails while daring greatly.

Theodore Roosevelt

Final Thoughts

Work like it all depends on you and pray like it all depends on God.

St. Ambrose

Have I done everything perfectly? Heavens no. I made plenty of miss-steps in the early days trying to find my way. Most clients, though, are understanding, flexible, and forgiving. If they don't come back because one time the table warmer wasn't high enough, or too high, send them a silent blessing and move on knowing other people are on their way to you at all times. Remember, there is more than one way to do everything, and there is no right or wrong for most things. Some ways just tend to produce more favorable results more often. Tell yourself it is okay when you do mess up. Allow yourself to make mistakes – most mistakes are not fatal. You will learn from them and continue to grow and improve. There were times when I was so distracted in a massage by outside thoughts that I could not remember if I had worked on both legs or just one. That was not a good feeling, I'll tell you!

Every experience is an opportunity to learn, grow, try new things, and achieve. The only true mistakes are experiences from which we fail to learn! My mantra for the first five years was a constant "I am getting better every day in every way". Keep your mind busy with a positive thought and there is no room or time for negativity. The Bible tells us in Matthew 17:20 that "If ye have faith as a grain of mustard seed, ye shall say unto this mountain, Remove hence to yonder place; and it shall remove; nothing shall be impossible." Every experience is a building block in the foundation of relationship. We are building relationships with our clients one experience at a time, and when we are honest about what doesn't go well, it helps our clients relate to us because they are just as human as we are!

Worrying about getting enough clients is a fear-based mentality. You are afraid of scarcity. Switch to believing in abundance and you will attract abundance. There are plenty of people in the city where you live, right? They all need massage, and those who are destined to come to you will do just that.

When I started massage school I had a vision of being a successful Licensed Massage Therapist. I saw myself using skills I would learn to help bring improved health to all of my clients. I visualized a busy practice and all the benefits that came with success. Today, many years after massage school and licensing boards, my vision has become a complete reality. Now I want to expand my vision to include success for you too. Our current "health" care system in reality operates as a sick care system. As massage therapists we promote health, prevention, and whole mind/body wellness, and I would love to see an increase in real health in our population.

We need more good massage therapists who understand their worth, have a passion for health and wellness, and who are successful at reaching potential clients and turning them into clients who feel good, enjoy life, and spend their money in fun and rewarding ways rather than on illness, medical procedures, and medications. Keep your vision in front of you every day and watch it take shape!

Whether you work for someone else or have your own practice, take care of yourself, treat your clients well, add excellence practices in every way, and you will quickly gain a following. Have faith that life unfolds exactly as it is supposed to. Love yourself, love your work, love life, do your best every day, and create more connections to others who will be drawn to you and to your loving and positive energy.

Once I realized that this is exactly where God wanted me to be, I knew I would succeed. He is behind me and guiding me all the way. My ideas are gifts from Him. When I'm inspired, I am "in spirit". The Higher Power is working in me and through me. There is no way I could have done this without His help. And if I can do it, so can you. "For with God all things are possible." (Mark 10:27)

Suggested Reading List

Accept No Mediocre Life by David Foster

EntreLeadership by Dave Ramsey

Getting to Yes by Fisher, Ury, and Patton

Love, Medicine, and Miracles by Bernie S. Siegel, M.D.

More Than Enough by Dave Ramsey

Rhinoceros Success by Scott Alexander

The Power of Intention by Dr. Wayne W. Dyer

The Bible

Who Moved My Cheese? by Spencer Johnson, M.D.

Your Erroneous Zones by Dr. Wayne W. Dyer

You'll See It When You Believe It by Wayne W. Dyer

About the Author

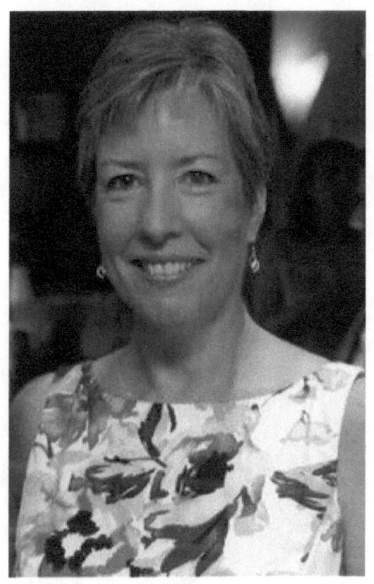

    Mary Alice Walter holds a bachelor's degree in psychology, graduated from SHI Integrative Medical Massage School in Lebanon, Ohio, and is licensed in Ohio and Kentucky. Self-employed as a Licensed Massage Therapist since 2005, she has mentored many new therapists along the way. Her basic philosophy in life is that we are all meant to serve each other in whatever way possible. This is her second published work, so far. Mary Alice lives in Northern Kentucky.

Index